STUDENT·NURSE·SERIES

Essential Paediatric Nursing

E. Fenella St J. Adamson   RGN RSCN RNT DN (Lond)

Formerly Senior Nurse Tutor,
Nottingham School of Nursing

Churchill Livingstone 🚢

EDINBURGH LONDON MELBOURNE AND NEW YORK 1987

CHURCHILL LIVINGSTONE
Medical Division of Longman Group UK Limited

Distributed in the United States of America by
Churchill Livingstone Inc., 1560 Broadway, New York,
N.Y. 10036, and by associated companies, branches
and representatives throughout the world.

First published 1987

ISBN 0-443-03628-4

British Library Cataloguing in Publication Data
Adamson, E. Fenella St J.
    Essential paediatric nursing.
    1. Pediatric nursing
    I. Title
    610.73'62   RJ245

Library of Congress Cataloging in Publication Data
Adamson, E. Fenella St J.
    Essential paediatric nursing.
    (Student nurse series)
    1. Pediatric nursing. I. Title. II. Series.
[DNLM: 1. Pediatric Nursing. WY 159 A221e]
RJ245.A32   1987   610.73'62   87-6596

Produced by Longman Singapore Publishers Pte Ltd
Printed in Singapore

Preface

This book is intended for RGN students as an introduction to the care of children, their everyday activities and their specific needs when they are ill. It also includes detailed information on child health in the community, and provides a brief summary of problems in developing countries.

The book may also be of value to nurse tutors for reference and as a source of discussion material, and to nursing staff and other professionals working with children in hospital.

How to use this book

The text is designed for use during the paediatric module in general training. Chapter 1 gives you an insight into what to expect and you will find reading the whole of Part One helpful before you start. Part Two provides more detailed information about the child's development, and family and community influences. The focus in Part Three is on practical care in health and sickness. Finally Part Four considers some of the wider social issues and future trends concerned with child health.

Acknowledgements

I am indebted to many friends and colleagues in Nottingham and Newcastle. These include Janet Campbell (mental handicap), Judi Harding (nursery nursing), Ros Lowe (health visiting), Jo Tatham (school nursing), Jeremy Watkins (dying), David Hull and Anne Nicholson.

My thanks also to Mark Brierley for his drawing and to Peter Swift who obtained it for me, also to Pip Edgar for help with the typing. For the front cover photograph I am indebted to Jacqueline and her mother, Lesley Thompson, Elizabeth Irwin and the photographer, Sylvia Grossick.

I am most grateful to Caroline Metcalfe-Gibson for the lively and detailed illustrations, to Carol Hull for her many helpful suggestions, and to David for his support and tolerance while I was unsociably preoccupied with the book.

Corbridge 1987   E. F. St J. A.

Contents

PART ONE   Introduction to the care of sick children

1. The nurse and the sick child   3
2. The child in hospital   17
3. Organisation of care   47

PART TWO   The child's background

4. The family   67
5. Development   89
6. Child health in the community   119

PART THREE   Practical aspects of children's care

7. A safe environment   143
   Body temperature
   Breathing
8. Communicating   180
   Playing
   School
9. Eating   205
   Drinking
   Eliminating

viii / *Contents*

10. Personal cleansing and dressing 238
    Mobilising
    Pre- and postoperative care
11. Dying 272

PART FOUR A wider view

12. Social problems 281
13. Trends in child health 292

Appendix Calculations relating to administration of drugs 308
Glossary 315
Index 323

PART | # ONE

Introduction to the care of sick children

Note

Throughout the text, the carer is referred to as 'she' and the child as 'he'. Also for convenience, 'mother' is used in many instances where father or mother would be equally appropriate.

The following terms are defined thus:

infant or baby   = under 1 year
toddler   = 1–3 years
pre-school child = 3–5 years.

The sick child
The student's
    background
The paediatric module
Historical background
The children's ward
    today
Observation of the sick
    child

1

The nurse and the sick child

What is different about nursing sick children? Surely they are small adults with similar needs, so nursing them should be much the same as nursing adults? This is a very common misconception. Although it is partly correct, there are major differences which pose an extra challenge and provide a bonus for those caring for children.

THE SICK CHILD

The child's anatomy and physiology differ in many respects from the adult's and these aspects often cause problems when he is sick. For instance the young child with an upper respiratory tract infection is more likely to develop an obstructed airway due to the small lumen of his air passages. An infection that might cause a mild attack of diarrhoea in an adult could lead to a severe attack of gastro-enteritis in an infant because his immunity is not well developed and he is more susceptible to fluid and electrolyte imbalance.

Equally relevant to the child's care is the degree of dependence of the child and the fact that he is developing emotionally, socially and intellectually as well as physically. This means that he has different needs at each age. His care has to be adapted accordingly, otherwise we are likely to hinder the child's normal progress at least temporarily, and at worst in the long-term too. Consider the following example:

Karen

Karen is a lively 14-month-old who comes from a happy home and has never been separated from her mother. Her progress to date has been normal, but Karen has just learnt to walk and her mother has noticed an unusual gait. The diagnosis of congenital dislocation of the hip is confirmed at the hospital outpatient department and Karen is now being admitted for treatment. Initially she has to lie in a head-down position with her legs in traction for at least 2 weeks.

This little girl now has several problems as well as the physical disorder. She is normally highly dependent on her mother not only for physical care but also for emotional security and therefore if her mother cannot stay with her, she will be unhappy and insecure. At 14 months she has just learnt to feed herself and is fiercely independent about this, but because of her position in traction, feeding herself will

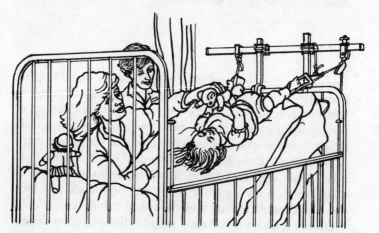

Fig. 1.1 Karen's position in traction.

be difficult. She strongly resists any attempt to help her. The challenge in caring for Karen is to treat her hip whilst at the same time preventing or reducing the adverse effects on her development and emotional stability.

THE STUDENT'S BACKGROUND

Many student nurses undergoing general training adapt very readily to nursing sick children. The student may already have experience in handling and caring for healthy children, brothers or sisters, or babysitting for family or neighbours. Some students may have done voluntary work with groups of children such as Brownies or in a home with the handi-capped. For others it may have been part of a child care or health studies course at school. Occasionally a student has worked as a nanny or trained as a nursery nurse. This is all useful experience prior to working in the children's ward but it is by no means essential. Students with no previous experi-ence whatsoever rarely have serious problems and usually adapt quite quickly. Those who are worried about dropping the baby while bathing him should relax. A student may wish she had three hands as the baby wriggles and kicks but she is unlikely to let him fall! All students can use their practical expertise already learnt in caring for adults, and those students who come to paediatrics reluctantly because they do not like children (not unusual) often surprise them-selves by enjoying the experience. Nursing children is demanding, but for most people it is also enjoyable and rewarding.

THE PAEDIATRIC MODULE

Whatever pre-conceived ideas or feelings the student may have, it is best to start the module with an open mind and a positive approach. Most nurses really enjoy it and their problem comes at the end when they do not want to leave. Child care is an important branch of nursing sick people as it provides useful information on health education, especially relating to the family. It is also valuable preparation for parenthood, possibly the most likely branch of child care with which you will be involved!

The first week of the module is probably spent in school. It is an introduction to the background knowledge on which children's care is based. Subjects include development, play, the child's normal environment and his needs, and how the hospital tries to provide for these when he is ill. Practical aspects are included and time may be spent in the ward where the student will work. Specific subjects, are included that may have caused concern previously to students, such as caring for a child having a convulsion or a child who has been abused. Another useful session is revision of arithmetic, required when calculating small volumes of drug solutions for children's doses.

The introductory week is therefore something of a 'first aid' course in how to survive in the children's ward when the student first starts. After a few weeks she will have settled in and will probably amaze herself by the confidence she has gained in a short time.

HISTORICAL BACKGROUND OF SICK CHILDREN'S NURSING

Changes in nursing care

Some student nurses will have had the experience of a stay in hospital as a child. When they are asked what they remember most vividly about this, they usually mention situations such as being nursed alone in a room, missing their parents or being attended by a horrible nurse! Less often they mention physical aspects of care like having to stay in bed. The emotional effects have often made a deeper impression than other aspects and research has confirmed the importance of meeting the emotional (or psychological) needs of children in hospital. If the students asked their mothers or grandmothers about similar experiences in their day, they would learn about stricter regimes with limited visiting of parents on certain days or possibly no visiting at all. In some instances parents were allowed to attend the hospital weekly at a set time to hand over gifts for the children and to observe them through a window, but not to talk to them. It was considered that seeing the parents made the children unhappy because they cried when the visitors came, and therefore it was not good for them. The staff were in complete control of the ward and the children. The parents had little or no say in what happened.

20th century developments

This type of rigid custodial care of children in hospital was the norm throughout the first half of this century, probably in line with care in general hospitals and children's homes. However, from the early 1900s, psychology developed as a subject in its own right. Freud and many others after him took a particular interest in the psychology of child development (developmental psychology). Gradually this led to a new awareness of children's needs and of the damage caused by separating children, especially younger ones, from their mothers or familiar caretaker. Research continues and Hall & Stacy (1970), for example, highlighted the child's social needs and the disruption caused by a stay in hospital. All these ideas have only been accepted and incorporated into nursing practice slowly. Practice still lags behind well-established theories of child care which best meet the child's needs. This slow progress explains why the nurses' and their mothers' experiences were different from what they see in the wards today. It also partly explains existing situations that do not entirely match up with accepted ideals of care.

Improving care

The earliest recommendations about improving the care of children in hospital were issued by the government in the 1940s and 1950s. The Platt Report (1959) was the first major report to stimulate action to improve emotional and other aspects of care beyond medical and nursing treatment. It recommended that children only be admitted to hospital if absolutely necessary and that they should be nursed in children's wards, separated from adult patients. Other recommendations included residential accommodation for mothers of under-5s, freer visiting, more facilities for children such as for play and schooling, suitably qualified staff and a child-orientated environment. Various government memoranda were subsequently issued at regular intervals which encouraged implementation of these recommendations, but change was painfully slow. The comprehensive Court Report (1976) reviewed the child health services in the United Kingdom and made further recommendations. Some of these have been implemented in a modified form in certain parts of the country.

Voluntary organisations have also contributed to improvements in sick children's care. The National Association for the Welfare of Children in Hospital (NAWCH) has been active since 1961 and is involved in helping children in hospital and their families. The most recent survey of children's wards carried out by the Consumers' Association in 1980 revealed that in spite of substantial improvements in many of the areas mentioned in the Platt Report, many of its recommendations have still not been implemented fully.

From children's hospitals to paediatric units

The sick child has traditionally been nursed at home by his mother, and for the vast majority of childhood illnesses this is true today. Even when children's hospitals were well established, sick children of rich families tended to be nursed by private nurses at home. The first children's hospital in the country was opened in Great Ormond Street, London in 1852. This was followed, during the second half of the 19th century, by the building of many others, usually in large cities. Several of these hospitals are in use today, for example in Derby and Edinburgh. Prior to this development, grouping of children in institutions, usually orphanages, had proved disastrous. Conditions were poor, caretakers were untrained and often unsuitable, infection was rife and the mortality rate was high with the result that most children died within the first few years of life. Following improvements in social conditions and advances in medical and allied sciences, from the 1880s onwards, children's hospitals and wards were found to serve a useful purpose and numbers of patients increased rapidly.

The present day

From these early beginnings our present situation has evolved. Sick children requiring hospital care are admitted to a

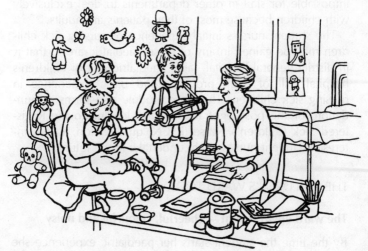

Fig. 1.2 A modern paediatric ward.

paediatric ward or unit of a distict general hospital, a children's hospital or the paediatric unit of a large teaching hospital. The district general hospital provides a valuable service near the child's home, while the children's hospital and large teaching hospital provide care for local children in cities, and specialised units for all children. The small children's hospitals are gradually being closed and the patients transferred to large paediatric units in vast modern hospital complexes. The children have benefited from this move in that modern and expensive facilities of laboratory, radiology and other departments are now close at hand. However, an invaluable part of the small hospital has been lost in the move — the total environment geared to children. The small building was less threatening and more friendly but even more important, every member of staff — nurse, porter, radiographer, doctor and laboratory technician and many more — all worked continuously with children and developed great skill in doing so. This made an ideal atmosphere for children and their families which is difficult to re-create in one part of a large modern general hospital. It is also impossible for staff in other departments to deal exclusively with children because most of their patients are adults.

The student nurse's initial experience of nursing sick children may be gained in any of these paediatric areas, that is in district general hospital, large paediatric unit or children's hospital. All of them provide good basic experience in nursing sick children. The basic module also forms a foundation for the post-registration course leading to the Registered Sick Children's Nurse (RSCN) qualification, which interested student nurses might undertake in the future.

THE CHILDREN'S WARD TODAY

The ward environment — cheerful, colourful and noisy

By the time the student starts her paediatric experience she will be accustomed to the appearance and atmosphere of adult wards—reasonably tidy, patients talking quietly to each other or resting silently, staff moving busily around. The children's ward is very different. At best it seems to be in organised chaos. It is noisy—babies are crying, children playing noisily together, the radio may be playing in the background or the television is on, or both! Every available surface seems to be covered with brightly covered pictures of every description, illustrated written work, posters, cards from family and friends and mobiles and collages made by the children themselves or with the schoolteacher's help. An architect of a new hospital was disappointed that the children's ward of his fine building could not be admired because every inch was covered with decoration!

The ward is certainly stimulating. Curtains and counterpanes are brightly coloured, often with well-known figures from children's stories which can be a great topic of conversation. In the treatment room there may be a picture on the

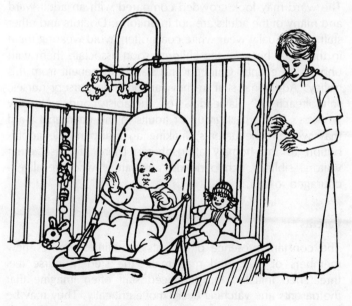

Fig. 1.3 Toys create a cheerful and friendly environment.

ceiling or a mobile hanging from it so that the child has something to look at when he is lying down on the couch. The babies are not excluded either, for colourful mobiles are hung above them and strings of toys tied across the cot. All these contribute to the overall impression of a bright, cheerful and friendly place.

Another surprise is that most of the children are up and dressed, running around the ward or in the schoolroom with the teacher. Many of the beds and cots are empty and it can be difficult to distinguish patients from brothers and sisters. Beware! They have been known to change places, the visitor may be trying the bed while the patient is playing underneath it. Identibands are therefore an essential safeguard for children.

The people

The ward may look crowded compared with an adult ward and many of the adults are not in uniform. Doctors and other staff who usually wear white coats often avoid wearing them in the ward because the children soon associate them with unpleasant events. Children and staff both benefit from this policy. Additional staff in the ward include nursery nurses, schoolteachers, playleaders or therapists and voluntary workers. The largest group of adults in the children's ward may well be the parents, making an indispensable contribution to the homely atmosphere. There are also other visitors, siblings, schoolfriends, and family who are all encouraged to visit.

Parents

The constant presence of parents sometimes worries new members of staff, and may make the student nurse feel threatened initially. Inexperienced staff often imagine that the parents are watching every move critically. They may be watching the nurse, but rarely do they criticise, and more often they are involved in the care with the nurse. Staff quickly come to enjoy the closer relationship with the patient's family and appreciate that the parents are the experts in their child's care and it is usually unwise to ignore their suggestions. Parents can teach the staff a lot about handling their child. Susan, a 14-year-old mentally and physically handicapped girl, could not swallow the tablets prescribed for a respiratory infection. The nurses tried various methods without success. Her mother knew what to do—the only way Susan could swallow tablets was by sucking them off a rubber teat.

More space is required than in most other wards for parents who are resident and also for those who visit all day. Resident parents need sleeping accommodation, bathroom facilities and a room where they can have a break from the ward and the child. Equipment of various sizes to suit all age groups requires more storage space which is rarely available.

Play

Play should be obvious in any area where there are children. It is an important part of their lives and a new activity for student nurses during working hours! There should be plenty of toys with opportunity and encouragement to play. A separate playroom provides space for adventurous play, for example with sand and water, in a life-size Wendy house or riding tricycles. Children play around each other's beds, on the floor or in bed. Do not be surprised to see a nurse sitting on the floor playing with a group of toddlers or playing trains under the beds in the ward. Some wards are lucky to have access to a garden, verandah or balcony for the children to play outside.

The student settling in

During the first day or two the student nurse may be aware of a lack of ward routine. Organisation of nursing care seems

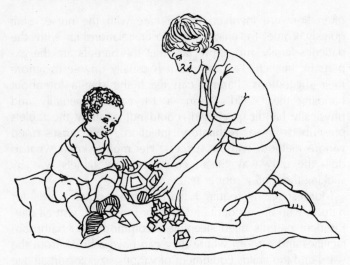

Fig. 1.4 Play can be hard work!

less structured than that to which she is accustomed. In fact this is intentional, the staff are working to make the ward as friendly and homely as they can. At the same time, of course, nursing care must be continued and essential tasks carried out punctually. It is easier to combine a relaxed atmosphere and efficient care when patient allocation is the method of organisation of work. Most students are accustomed to this method and it is well established in most paediatric areas.

Peaks and troughs in workload

The student will notice the rapid turnover of patients, many admitted for 24 or 48 hours only. The average length of a stay in hospital for a child is 3.5 days. The shorter the better for the child but it is hard work for the staff. The nurse returning from 2 days off duty has to get to know many new faces in the ward, several of whom will be discharged the next day. Another difficulty is the peaks and troughs in the workload which occur in most paediatric wards. It is impossible to control this because most of the admissions are emergencies and also children's conditions change for better or worse within a few hours. The new nurse may feel she lacks supervision at the busy times but finds the quiet times even more difficult. If there is no child whom she can help or play with, the student will probably be encouraged to read about the children's backgrounds in the notes or do some of her own work.

Slower pace

From the first day the nurse is likely to notice the slower pace of children's nursing. More time is taken gaining the child's confidence and procedures such as giving medicines take longer and cannot be hurried. Babies and young children, being totally dependent, require many hours of nursing time.

Infection is always a problem in children's wards because children contract more infections than adults and they are particularly vulnerable when sick. Handwashing and other measures to prevent cross infection are time-consuming but must be conscientiously carried out. Children who are at special risk of acquiring an infection in the ward, such as young babies, are usually nursed in cubicles. Likewise a child who is known to be infectious is isolated to protect the rest of the children.

OBSERVATION OF THE SICK CHILD

One of the most valuable skills for the nurse to develop while caring for children is accurate observation— developing the skill already learnt when nursing adults. A sick child requires closer observation because his condition changes so quickly and he cannot or is unlikely to tell the nurse that he feels different. If he is deteriorating, urgent action may be needed which requires prompt recognition of something amiss, usually identified by the nurse. Students in their first paediatric experience are not expected to become experts in this but they can make a useful contribution.

Martin

Nurse Brown was assigned to care for Martin aged 6 weeks for the second consecutive day. He was not seriously ill. This was only the nurse's first week in the ward but she managed well. Martin was feeding normally but during the 2 p.m. feed Nurse Brown thought he was somehow different though she could not explain why. She then paid close attention and noticed that intermittently he seemed to stiffen for a fraction of a second, and this was repeated at intervals. She did not know whether this was normal or not but she informed the ward sister at once. Martin was found to be having a type of fit which babies may develop, and appropriate treatment was started immediately. This prompt treatment controlled the fits and reduced the likelihood of them recurring. Martin was discharged home the following week, feeding well and gaining weight.

The nurse allocated to care for a child over a period of time is in the best position to notice any change in his condition. Nurse Brown was the only person who had observed a slight but important change in Martin's movements. Trained staff much prefer to be asked or to be told about anything the inexperienced nurse has noticed, even if it turns out to be unimportant, which it often will be.

REFERENCES AND FURTHER READING

Consumers' Association 1980 Children in hospital. A 'Which' investigation. Consumers' Association, London

Court S D M (Chairman) 1976 Fit for the future. The report of the Committee on Child Health Services. HMSO, London

Hall D, Stacey M (ed) 1979 Beyond separation. Routledge & Kegan Paul, London

Platt H (Chairman) 1959 The welfare of the child in hospital. Ministry of Health. HMSO, London

On admission
The family in the ward
Advice on visiting
Children's reactions to
    hospital and help
    given
Infants up to 7
    months

Older infants,
    toddlers and
    pre-school children
The schoolchild
The adolescent
Difficult situations in
    the ward

2

The child in hospital

Nursing the sick child means caring for the family. The first contact of the sick child with the hospital is through his parents and it seems natural and sensible to start with them.

ON ADMISSION

Parents entering the ward for the first' time are likely to be anxious about their sick child and probably over-awed by the hospital environment. The child may see his parents change from the confident adults he knows, who can answer all his questions, into hesitant people who feel that they are losing control of the situation and failing as parents when their child most needs them. The parents' uncertainty does not go unnoticed by the child whose own anxiety may be increased by this unusual behaviour. Most parents are re-assured when they realise that they are welcome in the ward at any time and can participate in their child's care. Once they have settled in and are fully involved, most parents quickly regain confidence.

When the child's admission is planned, details about

visiting and accommodation can be sent to the parents prior to admission. However most children are admitted to hospital as emergencies so no preparation is possible. Every family is warmly welcomed to the ward and during the initial chat with an experienced nurse, visiting arrangements and accommodation for parents are discussed. Although they are encouraged to stay, pressure is not put on parents who cannot or do not wish to. In no way are they made to feel guilty or neglectful.

Angela

Mrs Joan Evans was accompanied by her mother when she brought her 6-month-old daughter, Angela, to hospital with a chest infection. Angela was Mrs Evans' fifth child. One of her children had died as a baby, the two eldest had been taken into care because of neglect and Melanie, aged 2 years, lived with her grandmother. Mrs Evans had been married for a short time and subsequently lived with three other consorts. At this time she was living alone.

Mrs Evans was terrified of hospitals and resented all forms of authority which meant anyone in uniform. She would only come to hospital on condition that her mother came too. She was reluctant to speak to the staff and could not be persuaded to stay. Grandma was concerned about Angela and after a long discussion, they decided that she would stay in the hospital and that Mrs Evans would look after Melanie. The grandmother was a capable woman who was able to take over much of Angela's care and the baby benefited from her presence. When Angela was ready for discharge the health visitor was informed about her condition so that the family could be supported and supervised. In fact the health visitor knew the family well and although a lot of support was required initially, Mrs Evans coped fairly well and Angela made a good recovery.

THE FAMILY IN THE WARD

Resident parents

For the last 30 years children's wards have been encouraged, and from time to time instructed, to relax visiting rules and to encourage the presence of parents in the ward. It is UK government policy that all hospitals provide accommodation for parents of young children so that one of them can be resident with the child in hospital. It is the hospital's responsibility to inform the parents of this facility. The enthusiasm and sincerity of the ward staff when they suggest this option has been found to have more bearing on whether it is taken up than any official policy or ward notice.

Accommodation

Parents may be accommodated in a single room with the child, in a separate room in the ward or elsewhere in the hospital. Sometimes dormitory-type accommodation may be shared with several other parents. If necessary a camp-bed may be put up beside the child's bed and failing all else, the mother may opt to rest in a comfortable chair near the child rather than to leave him. The mother or father is offered whatever type of accommodation is available. A sitting-room is provided for mothers in the ward area where they can relax and make a snack if they wish. Resident parents usually eat in the staff dining room; those on supplementary benefit do not pay for meals.

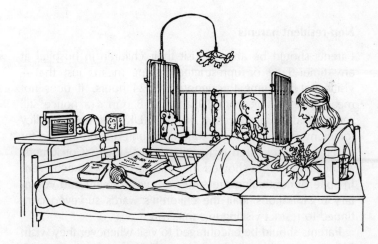

Fig. 2.1 Mother and child together — the ideal arrangement.

Advantages and disadvantages

The best arrangement, if it is possible, is for the young child to have his mother sleeping in the same room. She is immediately available, she is totally involved in his care and he has her comforting presence. The disadvantage for the mother is that she is likely to become very tired particularly if the nights are disturbed when the child requires essential nursing care. Parents do get very tired but they accept this as a small price to pay for being with their child. Nursing staff ensure that mothers have sufficient rest and also get breaks from the ward. A mother going out for an evening with her husband may seem to be taking advantage of the ward facilities, but a relaxing break in completely different surroundings may be just what she needs to keep her going. Nurses themselves find 8 hours in a ward long enough! Medication is occasionally prescribed for an exhausted parent who may be encouraged to go home for a good night's rest. Parents who are resident have the additional worry of leaving the family at home to fend for themselves.

Non-resident parents

Parents should be able to visit their children in hospital at any time. Free or unrestricted visiting means just that— visiting at any time throughout the 24 hours. It does not mean 'free visiting from 10 a.m. to 8 p.m.,' a notice still seen outside some wards. It has been UK government policy for many years that there should be unrestricted visiting for parents of all children in hospital, yet a survey (Consumers' Association, 1980) showed that this had not been achieved. In spite of continuing pressure from government and voluntary organisations, half the children's wards surveyed continued to restrict visiting in some way.

Parents should be encouraged to visit whenever they wish. Father may call in on his way to work in the morning or after an evening shift. If the parents have to choose between one long visit once a week or several short visits more frequently, the latter is preferable, because the child's link with his parents is not broken for so long. Visiting parents are involved in their child's care when they visit and, like resident parents, are considered as part of the ward team. Some parents are keen to stay or visit all day but are restricted by commitments at home.

Thomas

Thomas, aged 6 weeks, had been admitted to the ward because he was vomiting. Pyloric stenosis was diagnosed and he required surgery and a few days in hospital. His mother was undecided on whether to stay with him or to remain at home with her husband and the other children aged 3 and 6 years. She sought advice from the staff and after discussing it with her husband they decided that he would take a week's holiday so that he could look after the family while she stayed with Thomas.

In this instance the advantages of Thomas' mother staying were considerable, bonding between mother and baby would be maintained and Thomas would have the security of familiar handling by his mother. Babies of 6 weeks can already recognise the touch and smell of their mothers.

ADVICE ON VISITING

Nursing staff help parents by listening to their views and by explaining the advantages of visiting if this is required. They may be able to suggest alternatives which would enable a parent to visit more often or to stay with the child. Brothers and sisters may be brought along when mother visits and may occasionally stay too. Other family members may be able to help, either at home or by visiting or staying with the child. The family may need financial help with travelling expenses or they may have other problems for which the social worker's assistance may be offered.

Parents also worry about the child crying when they leave

after visiting. The nurse can explain to parents that although distressing, the child is expressing his feelings in his usual way, and that this is healthier than being quiet and withdrawn. They are advised never to leave the ward without telling the child that they are going and also to tell the child's nurse so that she can be with him. They can be reassured that most children settle quite quickly if they are left with a familiar nurse to comfort and distract them.

Henry

Henry, aged 2½ years, had been admitted earlier in the day to the children's ward for an operation the following morning. It was bedtime. He peered apprehensively from behind the grubby teddy which he was clutching. He stared at the strange surroundings in which he found himself. He felt alone, isolated in the cot which was not nearly as cosy as the double bed which he shared with his two brothers at home. Nothing was familiar except teddy who had been admitted with him. The strangeness was made worse because neither his mother or father were able to stay with him. The last he saw of his mother was as she waved goodbye and hurried out of the ward looking anxious. Henry was not sure whether his mother would come back. He had cried when she left but the nurse looking after him had comforted him, cuddled him for a while after which he settled and played half-heartedly, mostly just watching the other children.

Now at bedtime, tucked up in his cot, it was all too much and he burst into tears again. The nurse sat him on her knee, cuddled him and spoke soothingly to him. He soon calmed down so that the nurse was able to put him back in his cot where he fell asleep immediately, still clutching teddy.

CHILDREN'S REACTIONS TO HOSPITAL

Each child copes with admission to hospital in his own way depending on his personality, his background and his stage of development. Previous bad experiences related to hospital or separation from his mother in early life may have a detrimental effect on his attitude to hospital admission. Although children do not develop at the same rate, there are patterns of behaviour and reactions to a hospital stay which tend to occur at certain ages.

INFANTS UP TO 7 MONTHS

The young infant is not obviously distressed by being in hospital as he sleeps most of the time and seems to behave as he would at home. However the attachment of mother and baby to each other, which is called bonding, begins at birth or earlier and develops over a long period. Bonding is disrupted and may be adversely affected if mother and baby are separated. The mother may have difficulty re-establishing the previously close relationship with the baby. The baby, responding to his mother's feelings, senses her anxiety which in turn makes him unsettled. In any case his relationship with her has also been disrupted. A prolonged separation may contribute to long-term problems in the child's emotional development.

Most nurses enjoy looking after babies up to 7 months of age because they are co-operative (on the whole) and from a few weeks of age they respond happily to anyone. They smile and gurgle and feed well. However a study of behaviour of babies of this age, after discharge from hospital, suggested that they had not been totally unaffected. For the first day or two at home, they spent more time staring around the room and were less active than they had been before admission.

Helping the infant and his mother

A resident mother usually sleeps in the room with her baby and looks after him as she would at home. If she cannot stay she is encouraged to visit whenever possible. Bathing and feeding can be timed to fit in with her visits. A young mother may lack experience in handling and caring for the baby if he is the first born. She will need guidance and possibly instruction in practical aspects of care and reassurance in her handling of him. A lot of help can be given in informal conversation. If she lacks confidence it is advisable for her to take over his care completely for a few days before he is discharged, so that she gains confidence and reassurance that she can cope at home.

When the mother is unable to be present, the baby is cared for by one nurse for each span of duty in order to provide a mother substitute in a limited way. Even small babies have their likes and dislikes. Some settle better if they are placed prone in the cot, others will only sleep on their side. Some babies take their feeds unheated at room temperature, others prefer them warmed. A feed may be taken without a break for bringing up wind but most babies prefer one break and for some two or three may be essential. All babies take their feeds best when their preferences are taken into consideration. With continuity of care, one nurse can feed and care for the baby more effectively because she gets to know his individual ways and a relationship can develop between them.

OLDER INFANTS, TODDLERS AND PRE-SCHOOL CHILDREN

By the age of 7 months the child can discriminate between different faces. He recognises his mother and therefore misses her when she is absent, and is apprehensive about the attention of strangers. The toddler's main anxiety is separation from his mother and this intense attachment reaches its peak at about 2 years of age, after which it lessens gradually. Much has been written about the effect of hospitalisation and separation from parents. Robertson (1970) describes toddlers' reactions to hospital in three phases.

Protest. Firstly the child protests by crying. It may be loud and persistent. He is unco-operative and may struggle away from an unfamiliar person who is trying to comfort him. At least the noise draws attention to his feelings, he cannot be ignored for long and he gains the attention he needs. This phase may continue for a few days or several weeks.

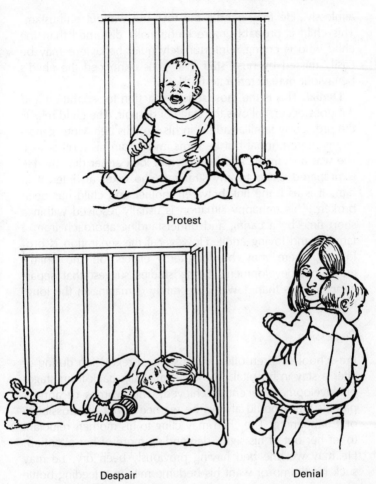

Protest

Despair

Denial

Fig. 2.2 Toddler reactions to hospital.

Despair. In the second stage the child ceases to protest. He does not cry so much and appears 'good'. The casual observer thinks that he has settled well but the reverse is true. He is quiet and withdrawn, and instead of playing normally, he sits watching other children or wanders around aimlessly. He may handle the toys but without enthusiam. This child is probably more emotionally disturbed than the child who is crying. Unfortunately quiet behaviour may be easily missed by busy staff. If it goes unnoticed the child's behaviour may deteriorate further.

Denial. This is the most serious reaction to separation and if it does occur, follows the stage of despair. The child rejects the previously familiar adults in his life. His behaviour generally is more normal but he turns away from his mother as if she was a stranger, and he does not look at her directly. He is prepared to go to any stranger who takes an interest in him. It is as if the link between mother and child has been broken. This unhappy situation is usually resolved within a short time by a caring and understanding approach from a familiar and loving adult. However if the separation is prolonged, there may be long-term effects on the child's emotional development. Some studies suggest that separations of less than 1 week are rarely damaging in the long-term.

Regression

Pre-school children often show signs of regression during or after a stay in hospital. The child may slip back from stages of development recently achieved. This worries or annoys parents who should always be warned about the possibility of it happening. The child may cling to his mother, reluctant to let her out of his sight, demanding more of her attention. He may wet the bed having previously been dry, he may suck his thumb or want his bedtime milk in a feeding bottle again. He may wake in the night, possibly with nightmares.

Helping the pre-school child

Mother's presence

The best method of reducing the effects of separation on the small child in hospital is to avoid it and for his mother to be resident throughout his stay. If she cannot do this, it will help the child if she can stay for a day or two to help him to settle into the ward. If neither parent can stay, a familiar family member may be willing to stand in for them. Non-resident parents are encouraged to visit as often as possible.

Patient assignment

When parents are not present, nurses care for the children using the system of patient assignment. One nurse looks after a small group of children carrying out all their care for a span of duty. Where possible, a child is cared for by the same nurse for several consecutive days. Thus the child relates to the minimum number of nurses and a closer relationship is possible with one nurse on each shift. As a result they act more effectively as mother substitutes when the parents are absent. Initially the nurse needs to spend time with the family getting to know them; preferably this starts with the admission procedure. She listens and talks to the child, and provides physical contact and security in caring for him, in cuddling and in play. Whenever possible the child's own nurse should be with him during unpleasant procedures such as taking blood, and for visits to other departments. All staff in children's wards need to understand the significance of children's behaviour. The observant nurse noticing a child who is very quiet, should stop and consider whether anything is wrong. Prompt attention may be required.

Advice for parents of children under 5 years

When the child is admitted, the parents should have the opportunity of discussion with a senior nurse so that problems or anxieties can be identified. The advice given to all parents is particularly important for the under 5s. They should never leave the ward after visiting without telling the child that they are going even if it upsets him, and they should also tell the child's nurse so that she can be with him.

Sometimes a mother may leave a glove or scarf to help the young child to understand that she is returning. Explanations about time should be adapted for the child's level of understanding. Small children understand 'when Daddy goes to work' better than '9 o'clock in the morning' and 'when you've had your tea' rather than 'later today'.

All parents should be warned that the young child may react to a stay in hospital after he has been discharged home, whether or not he appeared quite happy in the ward. They need to know that the best way to help the child is by giving him extra affection and attention. Parents should try to tolerate his temporary foibles without scolding or calling him babyish. They should understand that they will not spoil the child by doing this but will be helping him to work through this stage more rapidly.

THE SCHOOLCHILD

5–8 years

The 5-year-old normally goes to school each day so separation from home is not the problem it was for him when he was younger. However, he is still very dependent on his family and is likely to be anxious in a strange place like hospital without his parents. He has a lively imagination and his fears about what might happen in hospital may be his major concern.

Reacting to the strange environment, separated from home and unwell, he may well regress. For instance he may become attached to an old toy or blanket again or he may suck his thumb. He may want more of his mother's attention. He may have nightmares. He probably cries when he is frightened but has difficulty putting his fears into words. However, between 5 and 8 years of age, with increasing understanding and ability to communicate, most children settle quite happily if they are well supported by their parents.

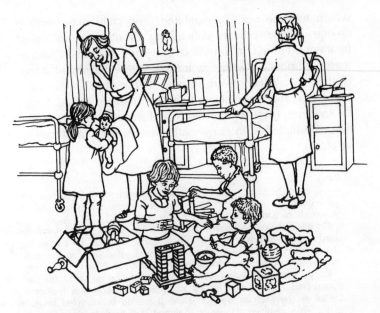

Fig. 2.3 5- to 8-year-olds happily settled in.

8–12 years

Now interests are increasingly centred outside the home, his friends become more important and he depends less on his family and home except as a base. For this reason, the child's major concern about being in hospital is usually the social disruption it causes. He is not too worried about being away from home although he needs parental support and enjoys visits from the family. He does miss his friends, the gang and their activities. One of the worst aspects of being a patient at this age is probably the restriction on physical activity. Being confined to bed on traction for 8 weeks or being in a wheelchair is hard for a normally active 10-year-old.

The child fears bodily injury but at the same time shows gruesome fascination in stitches, scars and parts removed, which may be proudly exhibited. The child may become anxious if he overhears staff talking about his condition or treatment. He may also misinterpret what he hears. Children tease and possibly worry each other with exaggerated stories of their own sufferings in hospital. Older children put on a brave face and are reluctant to admit to any fears which they try to hide. These hidden fears and frustrations may sometimes be hinted at in conversation or revealed in behaviour or play.

Barry

Barry, aged 12 years, was in hospital for treatment of leukaemia. He understood his condition and the need for unpleasant treatment, which previously he had seemed to accept philosophically.

On this occasion his behaviour changed. He rushed up and down the ward in his wheelchair at great speed doing 'wheelies' by tipping the chair back onto the large wheels. This was, of course, in the main thoroughfare of the ward, risking life and limb of all those in the vicinity.

Barry's uncharacteristic behaviour seemed to be an outlet for frustration and anger which he felt about his condition and treatment. Useful as this exercise was for Barry, it had to be curtailed because of the risks involved. However it alerted staff to Barry's true feelings so that they could give him the opportunity to discuss these. Together they might also devise an alternative activity which would be less hazardous.

Unusual or uncharacteristic behaviour may pass unnoticed by staff though it is likely to be spotted by parents who may comment on it.

Many children settle into hospital without difficulty and some really enjoy it. Others react by being blasé and over-confident or showing off. Some may be withdrawn and isolate themselves from other children. A child may be labelled 'difficult', he may be rude or resentful, or he may swear as he does at home. Children may form into a gang in the ward which may be beneficial in that they find mutual support and can help each other in a normal social grouping. On the other hand the situation can be difficult if children gang up against each other or exclude one child.

Helping the schoolchild

Contact with home

The young schoolchild benefits from his parents' daily visits. Fewer parents are resident with children over 5 years of age than with the younger ones unless there is a particular need. Sometimes a parent will stay for the first night or two until the child has settled. Visits of brothers and sisters and other members of the family help to maintain contact. Friends and schoolmates are always welcomed by school-age children: letters and cards are another reminder to the child that he is not forgotten. Consistent assignment of nurses to specific children over several days gives the child and his family more opportunity to build up trusting relationships with a few members of staff.

Homely environment

To reduce the strangeness of the ward, it is made as homely as possible (see Ch. 1). The newly admitted child and his parents are shown the layout of the ward and introduced to other children. Parents and staff, and the child if he is old enough, plan his care together and because parents are fully involved, the child's home routine is followed whenever possible. He wears his own clothes and is encouraged to consider the space around his bed as his, to decorate it with family photographs, and his own pictures, and to have some of his own toys. He can be involved in ward activities like helping to make his own bed or laying the table for meals. Sufficient toys for a variety of activities should always be available.

Reducing fears

Staff need to be alert to any unhappiness, regression or change in behaviour. Much of this will probably be due to unexpressed fears. A child may need help to talk about what

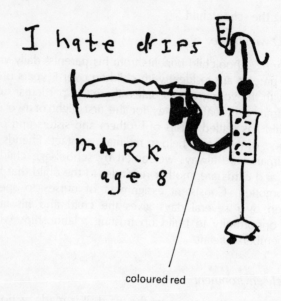

I hate dRIPs

mARK
age 8

coloured red

Fig. 2.4 Mark's feelings about intravenous therapy (by kind permission of Mark Brierley).

is worrying him and he is most likely to turn to his own nurse whom he trusts and with whom he has the closest relationship. He may be puzzled about his treatment, he may feel stupid wanting to talk about his fears, he may want to admit to feeling ill or miserable or he may want assurance about the outcome of his disease or the effect of his operation. Children may be helped by drawing a picture of hospital and then talking about it. Alternatively they might prefer to play doctors, nurses and patients. The nurse needs to take time listening to what the child is trying to say. He needs to know that he will be taken seriously. He may also be looking for reassurance that his illness is not a punishment for previous misdeeds or for telling his sister the previous week that he wished she was dead.

Truthful explanations

Roden (1983) found that 4- to 7-year-olds' anxiety during venepuncture was reduced by a realistic explanation beforehand. When truthful explanations are subsequently proved correct, the child gains confidence and the trusting relationship between nurse and child is built up. Parents are often the best people to explain things to the child. Sometimes they like the nurse's help in this. To be able to do this adequately, the parents require full information beforehand and to understand the child's condition, his treatment and anticipated progress.

Older children enjoy using technical terms; they pick up medical and nursing jargon quickly and enjoy confounding their friends with it. Children receiving long-term treatment learn about practical procedures that are part of their treatment, and have been known to correct doctors for a poor technique! Explanations for younger children require simpler, more homely words which they understand, for instance using the word 'tube' for a catheter.

Drawings and diagrams may be useful aids for a child of any age. Children may be shown equipment which will be used postoperatively and may handle it or practise using it beforehand. This is carefully planned and not shown to them if it might cause fear rather than reduce it. The child who understands his condition and treatment is less likely to be disturbed by what he overhears and will be able to correct the exaggerated stories of his friends.

Activity

All children in hospital who are well enough should be up and about, and dressed in day clothes. Most of those confined to bed can also be dressed in day clothes and lie on top of their beds. 8- to 12-year-olds have boundless energy and like to be occupied. School takes up most of the day in hospital and outside these hours some energetic games are useful. Even for those confined to bed, games can be devised using bean bags or balloons. Team games and group activities are usually popular.

A good example of a social activity in the ward which children enjoy is to have a tea-party. One or two children can send out invitations to a few selected people, for instance staff and fellow-patients. They can make a postbox to receive the replies. On the appointed day they can help to make the sandwiches and bake small cakes in the ward kitchen. Those confined to bed can decorate bought cakes. Then all the children can enjoy the party.

Children should be helped to make their stay in hospital a positive experience in which they mature a little and gain confidence. They may become more self-reliant, and find themselves able to cope with unpleasant situations which they would rather avoid. School work can progress, new skills may be learnt, and new friends made.

THE ADOLESCENT

Adolescence begins at puberty and is usually considered to end around 18 years of age. Young adolescents are usually admitted to children's wards, as are some older ones with long-term illness who benefit from the continuity of care provided by the familiar paediatric team. Rapid growth during the teens often necessitates frequent adjustments to treatment. Older physically and mentally handicapped teenagers may also be admitted to paediatric wards for medical treatment or surgery. The effects of long-term illness, disability, and disease which shorten life, are mentioned in this section because they are the problems which some teenagers have to face.

Loss of dependence

For the adolescent, developing from child to young adult, the loss of independence associated with being a hospital patient is a considerable drawback. He may tolerate this stoically and with good humour or may hide his feelings. He is more likely to react either by regressing to become dependent and demanding, or by being rebellious, difficult and moody. One minute he may be rude and critical of parents or staff for being too strict and treating him like a child, the next he is in tears and in need of sympathy and support. Minor incidents can result in outbursts of temper and demands to be left alone.

The normal if stormy adjustments which occur in the relationship between the adolescent and his parents may be disrupted when he becomes a patient. The teenager may blame his parents for his disorder or for bringing him into the hospital unnecessarily. His parents may become more protective and authoritarian in their anxiety, for instance they may insist on supervising or even carrying out the treatment which he should be doing for himself.

Social isolation

Problems can arise if the teenager is the only one of his age in the ward. His normal group of friends provide daily support at home and are usually happy to visit. However they may lack the experience and insight to be able to give him the extra support he needs as a hospital patient. He may also feel inferior, and distance himself from them, feeling unable to relate on equal terms in his disadvantaged situation. Without suitable leisure facilities and companions with similar interests he can easily become bored.

Body image

The young adolescent girl's heightened awareness of her body makes her shy and often acutely sensitive about exposing her body. Most are embarrassed about undressing in public and hate any physical examination which might involve undressing. The typical consultant's ward round when several pairs of eyes are fixed on the patient in bed is the adolescent's (and many adults') nightmare. All adolescents are sensitive to criticism about their appearance and become anxious about the slightest defect. Boys want to be tall and manly and are anxious if they are small or not growing as quickly as their friends. Girls are more worried about spots and scars, anything which mars their beauty. The shock for the adolescent who is told that he or she requires disfiguring surgery such as amputation, or cytotoxic therapy with the resultant alopecia, is understandably devastating.

Other problems

The adolescent may be keen on maintaining a high level of physical fitness in spite of or because of his disease or disability. While in hospital a boy might be concerned about whether he will be in the cricket team next term. The girl may worry that her diabetes will affect her performance in athletics in which she excels. The sedentary life of a hospital patient and the lack of training may result in a loss of confidence as well as fitness so that the adolescent becomes despondent and depressed.

School work may suffer. The adolescent may find it difficult to concentrate in the ward or when he is not feeling 100%. Therefore preparation for examinations may suffer, if indeed he is well enough to take them. Those with long-term disorders or a shortened life expectancy may find it difficult to apply themselves and easily become depressed. They may wonder if the effort put into academic work is worthwhile and how their condition will effect their chances of finding a job. After a long stay in hospital or a serious illness, the adolescent may become institutionalised and be uneasy about leaving the security which the hospital provides.

Medical treatment continued at home for prolonged periods or for life is a likely cause of rebellion and non-compliance. As a result the youngster occasionally requires hospital treatment. A diabetic may be admitted in a precomatose state after a feast of chocolates, or a boy recovering from a head injury may be admitted having had a fit because he failed to take his anti-convulsant tablets regularly.

Helping the adolescent

Independence

If a purpose-built adolescent unit is not available, the needs of young teenagers are best met in the children's ward. Staff are geared to the requirements of varying age groups, and facilities for unrestricted visiting and regular schooling are beneficial. Whatever the type of ward, adolescents need an area which they can call their own. This often has to be a double room with another teenager, a bay or section of a

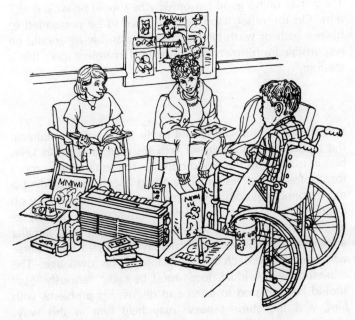

Fig. 2.5 Helping to promote group feeling among adolescents.

ward with several patients of the same age or failing all else, a single room.

Although adolescents (boys and girls) enjoy helping with the small children in the ward, they do not appreciate living in the same area. They require privacy. Ideally they should also have their own day room for which they are responsible. It can be suitably decorated with posters of their choosing and furnishing with hi-fi and other essentials. In this way they are accepted as a separate group and can entertain their friends in their own environment. This encourages a group feeling and a greater sense of identity.

Ward regulations should be minimal and the reasons for any essential rules should be explained. If the teenager is well enough he should have permission to come and go, for instance for walks or to spend weekends at home. The adolescent should be involved in planning his own day. There may be no good reason why he should be woken at 7 a.m. On the other hand he may have to be persuaded to have a bath or wash his hair. Where possible he should be responsible for his own basic care, and treatment too if this is feasible.

Social contacts

Friends are encouraged to visit freely. They help to maintain the adolescent's relationship with his own group and keep him in touch with the world outside. The separate day room for adolescents is less inhibiting and useful in providing a more normal environment where visitors and patients are on a more equal footing. The adolescent may turn to his parents for support, sometimes he may prefer to talk to a familiar adult or to a member of staff. He may choose a student nurse who seems approachable and close to his own age. The adolescent's individual needs must be taken seriously. Staff should be prepared to listen and discuss his problems with him, and the student nurse may help him in this way. However should she find that she is unable to help him with complex feelings and anxieties, the nurse should tell a senior member of staff. Specialist help is sometimes required. Female student nurses will realise that older adolescent boys near their own age may be attracted to them and may try to take advantage of their situation in hospital.

Respecting feelings and helping body image

The sensitive feelings of young people should be respected. Complete privacy is required for the teenager who has to undress; screens should be adequate and correctly placed, curtains fully drawn so that there are no gaps. Unnecessary exposure of an adolescent during physical examination or nursing procedure should be avoided. Patients should not be expected to talk about their symptoms, feelings or personal problems where other people can overhear the conversation.

Boys who are concerned about their short stature which is due to delayed puberty caused by certain chronic conditions can be reassured that they will grow eventually. Others may need help to come to terms with the fact that they will always be small. For girls, general advice can be given about skin care. It is helpful to the patient before an operation to demonstrate the site and length of the scar and to explain how it will look immediately afterwards and subsequently.

Additional support/help

All adolescents attend the hospital school daily, some more enthusiastically than others, though there is usually no reluctance among those who are working for examinations. Extra tuition may be possible for them and examinations can be taken in the ward if necessary. Discussion and encouragement is often required for those with chronic disease, a handicap or shortened life expectancy.

Little help is available for the teenager who wants to keep fit. Physiotherapy may be part of his treatment, for instance after a fractured tibia. In some hospitals it may be possible to use the physiotherapy department's swimming pool or gym.

Helping parents

Parents may find the problems of their adolescent offspring even more difficult when he is in hospital. Staff should explain that his behaviour in the ward could be due to the anxieties discussed above, which parents may not have appreciated fully. They may need help to support the adolescent without being overprotective. The adolescent who rebels against long-term treatment may be more prepared to discuss this with professional staff than with his parents. It is important that both parents and patient fully understand his condition and its treatment. Parents of the younger adolescent may need to supervise discreetly while letting him be responsible for all his own treatment. By the late teens he should be independent if his treatment allows.

DIFFICULT SITUATIONS IN THE WARD

Discipline

Discipline is occasionally a problem in the children's ward. One of the difficulties is that the children are accustomed to a different style of control at home. This varies from a rigid code of behaviour and manners to no control whatsoever. A certain amount of discipline is desirable for children and also for the smooth running of the ward. Setting limits of acceptable behaviour gives the young child security, for he may be frightened of his strong emotions which he cannot yet control. The older child needs help towards self-discipline.

Preventing troublesome behaviour

Prevention is easier than coping with bad behaviour. The ward sister and trained staff set the standards of acceptable behaviour within the ward. These should be loyally maintained by all staff so that the children can see that any rules are fairly maintained and that punishment, if necessary, is consistent. Children are quick to assess a situation and the people controlling it and will react accordingly. Apparent bad behaviour in the ward is often due to the child's anxiety or fear about his situation rather than to naughtiness. Giving the child time to talk and listening to any anxieties he has, may well resolve the problem.

Threats and punishment

Unacceptable behaviour requires firm handling. Ideally punishment is appropriate for the misdeed, given as near to the event as possible, is fair, and afterwards the whole incident forgotten. Punishment in the ward is more difficult because of the numbers of staff and the ease with which one nurse can be played off against another. Any threats of punishment should be enforceable but this is easier said than done. The nurse who forbids a child to watch his favourite television programme later in the day may well have gone off duty and forgotten to tell anyone. In any case the child is in a ward with several other children who are watching the programme. However, when a child ignores warnings he should be punished. A nurse should never smack a child or even give him a tap on the hand with a hairbrush, for disciplinary action may be taken against this nurse on the grounds of patient assault. Married nurses who are used to disciplining their own children may find this extremely difficult, but they must comply with this rule. Situations where parents are sitting beside the child who is behaving badly and not controlling him, are particularly trying. The nurse can enlist the parents' help, reason with the child or be firm with him. If she is frustrated or desperate she should ask another member of staff to take over and leave the situation.

Fair play

It is quite common for children to hit each other in boisterous play but in the ward it may need to be controlled. If the

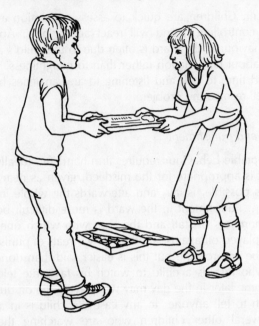

Fig. 2.6 Disputes require tactful handling.

situation is getting out of hand, the two parties should be separated, both points of view heard and a decision made which will probably be a compromise. Children respond to being treated as individuals, and to their views being heard and respected when decisions have to be made. Boredom can be a cause of bad behaviour. Sometimes it is best to change everybody's activity and start again. Older children may be troublesome when they form gangs. It helps to find out who is the leader and then try to enlist his help or find out his problem as he will be enciting the others.

Any child is likely to become unco-operative and difficult if his play is suddenly disrupted by an order to go and wash his hands for lunch or to put all his toys away immediately. Children should be warned about 15 minutes beforehand that they are going to have to stop what they are doing. This gives them some control over their own situation and allows them to conclude their activity in a more satisfactory way. Children, just as much as adults, should have an explanation for any request that is made. If the nurse cannot explain the reason to the child she may ask herself if there is one.

Temper tantrums

Tantrums in the toddler age group are normal but in the middle of a busy ward they are difficult to ignore. They occur when a child is frustrated and thwarted in what he wants, when he has not yet developed self-control and is too young to understand a simple explanation. Ideally a known adult whom the child likes should handle the situation. The child should be removed from the scene and taken to a quiet spot which in the ward usually has to be his cot, the curtains may be drawn around him but he should not be left alone.

After the initial anger has died down he is usually ready to be picked up and cuddled but the rage may last for several minutes and persist through several overtures to comfort him. It is important for the adult to remain unruffled, and for the toddler to feel by the adult's response that he is still loved, although this particular behaviour is unacceptable. He will gradually settle and may go back quietly to his previous activity or he may prefer an alternative.

Nightmares

Nightmares are common both in hospital and after discharge particularly when the child's illness or treatment has been frightening or painful, for instance after a major operation or an accident. Comfort and the presence of a reassuring person are essential. The child may feel better if a light is put on or he may be more comfortable in the dark. Probably younger children are more affected, but a child at any age should be attended to immediately he awakes crying. Some children cannot put their fear into words, while others will want to explain the whole dream before they are reassured. A warm drink, making him comfortable, staying with him for a while and possibly leaving a light on are all measures which help the child to settle to sleep again.

The death of a child

The greatest fear for most new students about nursing children is that of a child dying in the ward or having to care for one who is terminally ill. This brief introduction may allay some of these very natural fears. The subject is discussed in more detail in Chapter 11.

Reactions to a child's death

The nurse worries about her reactions to seeing a dying child, her distress and how she will cope with it. She wonders how she will respond in the situation and if she will be able to help the child and his family. Everyone feels like this initially and it is widely accepted that the death of a child is more difficult and distressing than the death of an adult. One possible reason for feeling this way, which applies to many students, is that the nearer one is in age to the dying person the more distressing it usually is. Older married students with families may associate closely with the parents who are nearer their own age. It is a very emotional situation too because of the idea of an unfulfilled life and the unfairness that the small body has had such a short life.

Sharing the sadness

When a child dies the staff are fully involved with the parents who may have been living in the ward for some time and with whom they have a close relationship. The old idea of the stiff upper lip and the nurse not showing any feelings is out of date. Staff can have similar feelings about the dying child as the parents, that is sorrow, anger and grief. It is quite acceptable to show sorrow and sadness and to share it with the parents. In fact parents often say afterwards how they were helped by seeing the doctor or nurse crying with them.

Putting feelings into action is often the most helpful way of relieving these feelings. The nurse can do this in caring for the child and supporting the parents. Being willing to stay in the situation with the family, and responding to what is happening at the time, shows a caring and sensitive attitude more effectively than words can. No forced or special conversation is necessary.

Support for staff

Trained staff in paediatric wards are well aware of the effects of a child's death on other staff particularly on inexperienced nurses. Any problems or specific anxieties of an individual nurse can be identified before she is introduced into the situation. The student does not work in isolation but is supported by a trained member of staff who shares in the family's care. Group discussions in the ward may be arranged and provide an opportunity for airing feelings and discussing difficulties. Staff who work permanently with terminally ill children find the work stressful at times but also challenging and rewarding.

Postscript

The incidence of deaths in children's wards generally is not high and most student nurses will complete the paediatric module without a death occurring in the ward where they are working. In a few specialised wards the likelihood of a child dying is greater than normal, either because children have specific diseases for which there is no cure, or because high risk surgery is carried out on children whose lives are threatened by their disorder. In these areas special help is available for staff who require support.

REFERENCES AND FURTHER READING

Consumers' Association 1980 Children in hospital. A 'Which' Investigation. Consumers' Association, London

Douglas J W B 1975 Early hospital admission and later disturbances of behaviour and learning. Development Medicine and Child Neurology 17(4): 455–480

Hall D, Stacey M (ed) 1979 Beyond separation. Routledge & Kegan Paul, London, ch 8

Hawthorn P J 1974 Nurse—I want my mummy. Royal College of Nursing, London

Jolly J 1981 The other side of paediatrics. A guide to the everyday care of sick children. Macmillan, London

Robertson J 1970 Young children in hospital. Tavistock, London

Roden J 1983 Will this hurt? Royal College of Nursing, London

The ward team
  Nursing staff
  Parents
  Nursery nurse
  Schoolteacher
  Liaison health visitor
  Playleader

Planning the sick child's
  care
The nursing process
  Assessment
  Planning
  Evaluation

3

Organisation of care

THE WARD TEAM

Many people are involved in caring for a child whilst he is in hospital. The members of the team will differ depending on the child's problems but will usually include the following people who would not be part of the ward team in an adult ward.

Nursing staff

The qualification for registered nurses who specialise in the care of children is the Registered Sick Children's Nurse (RSCN) certificate. Over 90% of sisters in charge of paediatric wards have this qualification and all staff who intend to care for sick children are advised to gain this certificate.

In hospitals where the RSCN course is undertaken, general student nurses work alongside RSCN students in the children's department. These students are taking either a post-registration course, a basic RSCN course in Scotland, or a combined training for RGN/RSCN. Although some post-registration students have had considerable experience as trained nurses, they are usually considered as senior students in the ward team. This enables them to make the most of the limited time which they have on the course, and to concentrate on developing practical skills in caring for children, without additional management responsibility.

One aspect of nursing children which is new to general nurses is that of making parents welcome as members of the ward team and helping them to become fully involved in patient care.

Helping the parents

With parents constantly in the ward it is easy for staff to assume that they know or should see what they can do. This is not always so. Parents need help from nurses to understand how they can participate in the child's care. On the one hand they do not always realise what information the staff need to know about their child and on the other they often wait for instructions from nursing staff before daring to do anything. The nurse helps the child's family to feel at home in the ward, and finds out how much the parents would like to do for their child. Initially they require an explanation about everything just as new trainees do, for instance where they can find equipment, how to use it and how to dispose of soiled clothing and rubbish. Then they may require instruction on specific procedures such as wearing a gown correctly. The nurse should explain exactly how much they can do, and tell them of any restrictions and any ward areas from which parents are excluded, for which a reason should be given. She should help the parents initially when they are caring for the child and always be ready to step in if needed. If parents are uncertain they should be encouraged to ask for help. All parents including those who seem very capable, require support and reassurance that they are doing well. The observant nurse watches for signs of tiredness and strain and does not leave parents for too long without offering help. They may also need encouragement to look after their own health and the nurse can suggest a break or some refreshment.

Parents

The mother's role in the ward team is described here. It could equally well be the father's, or the parents may share the care, taking it in turns to stay with the child.

Giving the child security

The mother's presence in hospital gives the young child a security which he cannot gain from any source other than a

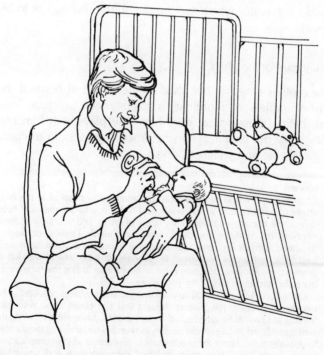

Fig. 3.1 A familiar face provides security.

familiar caretaker. Security and support is provided in normal mothering activities as well as during less pleasant and sometimes painful procedures, providing the mother wishes to be present. Her familiar touch in everyday care gives the child confidence.

Interpreting the child's needs

The young child's mother protects him from a strange world which would otherwise create many difficulties for him. The mother is the expert in understanding her baby's cry or her toddler's own special language and his frustrations. She can predict his reactions and anticipate his needs. Parents of older children will be able to recognise changes in their child's behaviour which may be due to the situation or to his illness.

Daily care of the child

The mother cares for her child as she would at home if she wishes, unless extraordinary circumstances preclude this. She baths, dresses and feeds him. She plays with him and may carry out technical nursing procedures after instruction, if she is able and willing to do so.

Edward

Edward was 6 weeks old when he was admitted to hospital in the early stages of heart failure, which was found to be due to a congenital heart defect. He became cyanosed after bouts of crying and was slow to feed. Although his condition improved rapidly with medical treatment, feeding remained difficult for he would only take about 30 ml of milk at each feed. The remainder was given by nasogastric tube which was left in position. His mother took over most of his care including the tube feeds, once she had been taught the procedure.

Quite soon Edward was fit to go home but one problem persisted—his reluctance to feed. His mother thought that she could cope with tube feeding at home although she had never passed a nasogastric tube. As the staff considered her a suitable person to take this on, she was taught how to pass the tube, about the precautions to be taken and the complications which might arise. Instruction included demonstration and supervised practice after which she continued to practise unsupervised with occasional checks by staff.

As soon as she was confident, mother and baby were discharged home. The district nurse would call regularly and Edward's mother could telephone the ward if she was worried.

Edward thrived at home although he required tube feeding for a further 2 months. His two older sisters were thrilled to have him back and his parents were equally pleased to have a normal family life again. Major surgery would be performed to correct Edward's heart defect when he was older.

Teaching practical skills to parents and children is an integral part of nursing sick children. It might involve any procedure from testing urine to nasopharyngeal suction.

Most parents are happy to help at mealtimes, to give bedpans, to chart fluid intake and output, and to collect urine specimens. Many also prefer to be present during painful procedures such as taking blood specimens or the dressing of a wound. They are invaluable in supporting the child and may also help in some procedures. Anxious mothers who find it too distressing may prefer to stay outside, ready to comfort the child afterwards. The mother decides what she wants to do, the nurse supports and may give advice.

Parents can also provide background information about the child which may have been omitted from the admission history, for instance how best to settle the child if he wakes at night. When a parent is involved in planning the child's day, his home routine is disrupted as little as possible. Parents not only care for their own children but often help others whose parents are not present. A mother may supervise a group of children playing, read a bedtime story to a restless child or act as a mother substitute to another child. Parents help each other in the ward. They are suffering similar strains and stresses, they have opportunities to share their anxieties and thus provide valuable support for each other.

Advantages and disadvantages for resident parents

Close relationships inevitably develop between staff and parents who work together for any length of time. This is beneficial for both groups and for the sick child. One of the resident parents' greatest problems is boredom. Remaining in one room with one child for several days is trying in the extreme. Meadows (1969) describes these feelings and the 'Which' Report (1979) found that 70% of resident parents were bored and 33% very bored.

Resident parents and those who visit all day benefit by being present when the doctor examines the child. The mother is kept right up to date with the child's progress and treatment, she can ask questions and may be involved in discussion about the child. She usually has a good grasp of the child's treatment and is proficient in practical aspects of care. She is therefore able to continue this at home if it is required, which may mean that the child can be discharged sooner than would otherwise have been possible.

A positive result of parents caring for their sick child in hospital is that they gain confidence in their role as parents. Instead of feeling that they have failed their child when he most needed them, they realise that they have played an important part in his recovery. Parents may also have learnt new nursing skills in the process; they may have lost long-standing fears of hospital and may have picked up useful hints on child care or other health topics.

Nursery nurse

The nursery nurse is skilled in caring for young children and can be a great help and support to student nurses during their paediatric experience. Nursery nurses are usually employed as playleaders and in this role they are not involved in nursing care. Some may be employed to help with the child's everyday care but this does not include technical nursing procedures. The nursery nurse acts as a mother substitute, providing consistent care for young children when parents are unable to visit. She is readily available in the ward, not distracted by other duties nor associated with painful procedures.

A qualified nursery nurse has undertaken a 2 year training and gained the Certificate of the National Nursery Examination Board. The course covers child development and the total care of the child from birth to 7 years. As well as learning theoretical aspects, the students gain practical experience in day or residential nurseries, nursery and infant schools, hospitals and homes for handicapped children.

Schoolteacher

The teacher and hospital school maintain a link with home life by providing a familiar routine and similar work. When the child is admitted, the hospital teacher contacts the child's school to find out what his class is doing, so that the same work, sometimes the same books, can be given. At the same time the teacher will learn about any difficulties which the child has, and she may then be able to give individual help or, if appropriate, report the problem to the medical staff. On the other hand the ward doctor may ask the teacher for her opinion about the child's intellectual ability, his attitudes to school or any behaviour problems observed.

The child may benefit from the closer contact with the teacher which is possible in hospital. He may choose the teacher as confidante because he spends more time with her than with any other member of staff and she is not involved in his treatment. The hospital teacher needs to be sensitive to the children's feelings and aware of the possible effects of illness and hospitalisation. She also needs to be adaptable so that she can adjust to each child's needs in order to provide suitable work for a wide range of ages and abilities. Teachers who work in hospital have all had experience in ordinary

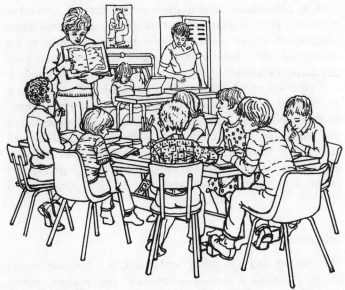

Fig. 3.2 School in the ward.

schools and are employed by the Local Education Authority. The head teacher is responsible for the day-to-day running of the school.

Liaison health visitor

The liaison health visitor (LHV) acts as a link between hospital and community. She may be based in either place though usually in the latter at either a health clinic or a surgery, where she may have a small case-load. Her main responsibility is to maintain good communications between community staff and the ward in order to ensure continuity of care throughout the child's illness. The LHV and the ward sister work closely together; they are in contact with each other on most days either by telephone or when the LHV visits the ward.

The ward doctor may ask the LHV for information about

the background of a child in the ward, the family situation or a specific social problem. The LHV then contacts the family HV and possibly other agencies too, and reports back to the doctor. Much of the work of the LHV is related to the discharge of children from hospital. If any treatment or supervision is required after discharge, the LHV again contacts the family HV and any other staff who will be involved. She gives them the details about the child's care and ensures that they have all the information they need to ensure a smooth transfer from hospital to home care.

Playleader

The playleader may work anywhere in the hospital where there are children, for instance in any type of children's ward, in the outpatients department or in special units such as those for handicapped children. Her aim is to encourage the children to play and to enable them to do this by providing a relaxed, secure but stimulating environment and a wide range of activities. The child may be isolated in a cubicle. He may be one of a group in the ward or he may be mobile and able to play in the playroom or out of doors.

The child may need help in his choice of activity, and encouragement to join with other children in a game. Supervision may be necessary to see fair play in a group. The playleader chats to the children and encourages them to talk to each other. She encourages their own ideas and provides opportunities for hospital play. She often contributes to the child's recovery by providing an activity for a specific purpose such as a game which involves a child using his partially paralysed hand.

Playleaders are usually nursery nurses, infant teachers or people who have had considerable experience working with children. Others have completed a course for playleaders and some health authorities make this a prerequisite for all staff taking up these posts. All those who care for children should be able to act as playleaders when necessary.

PLANNING THE SICK CHILD'S CARE

Planning begins when a decision is made that the child requires hospital care. Alternatives to hospital admission include day care in hospital, or home nursing provided by a paediatric home nursing service. The child benefits from these schemes but they are only appropriate for treating certain disorders, and the suitability of the home conditions is usually assessed beforehand. With good planning, these services can be safe and effective.

Day care

Many minor operations, and investigations with or without anaesthetic, are carried out on a day basis. The child arrives at the hospital, partly prepared for operation, and after a check-up to ensure that he is fit, receives the normal pre- and postoperative care. In some areas, children with medical problems, such as a child with a moderately severe asthmatic attack who is not seriously ill, may be treated in the children's casualty department or paediatric ward. Treatment and observation are continued throughout the day and the child is often well enough to go home in the evening. The mother is encouraged to stay with the young child throughout his day in hospital.

Paediatric home nursing service

The number of these schemes is small and each one is organised slightly differently though they have much in common. The staff are usually trained district nurses with the RSCN qualification. The team is based either in the local paediatric unit or in the community but all staff are in close touch with the paediatric hospital services.

Children nursed at home may be suffering from a variety of disorders ranging from acute infections to terminal care requiring oxygen therapy. In some areas specialist health visitors provide valuable practical help and counselling for specific groups of clients, for example families with a handicapped or a diabetic child.

THE NURSING PROCESS

The nursing process is widely used as a method of organising care logically and systematically. To be effective it should be based on a nursing model suited to the particular group of patients involved.

Certain concepts in Orem's model of nursing are appropriate to children's care. In considering the patient's need for self-care, she describes the patient at a certain point between the extremes of complete dependence and total self-care, and writes about the nurse providing a 'developmental environment'. This meets the needs of the child with his changing levels of dependence. Orem also emphasises family involvement in the patient's care, and her description of the nurse's role in assisting patients is equally appropriate for nurses helping the parents of sick children.

The Roper/Logan/Tierney nursing model can be adapted to patients of any age group. It is based on a model of living, and uses activities of living as a framework for the nursing process.

The nursing process is familiar to most nurses. Assessment, planning and evaluation are discussed here and implementation of care is described in Part Three.

Assessment

The assessment begins when the child walks into the ward with his parents for the first time. The impression of a shy apprehensive 8-year-old holding his mother's hand, or alternatively lagging behind his parents because he has been studying the pictures in the corridor en route, says something about each of them.

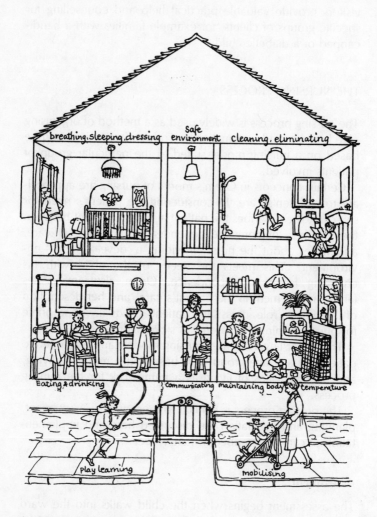

Fig. 3.3 Activities of living.

Listening to the child and his family as well as picking up non-verbal clues provide information about an individual. The interaction of family members with each other is relevant, for it affects the child. Assessment is not a single procedure or document but a continuous process which is made more complete as more is learnt about the patient. The child's own assessment of his condition should be included as well as his parents' views.

Taking the nursing history

The admission procedure is made as informal as possible (see Ch. 2) and if possible, organised so that the nurse admitting the child will continue to be his nurse for the next few days when she is on duty. Before starting it is helpful, if possible, to read the family doctor's letter and scan the medical notes. These give useful information such as parental illness or a previous cot death which might affect how the nurse approaches the parents. The parents and nurse should be sitting comfortably during this initial conversation, while the child may choose to join in, to play with toys nearby or to sit on his mother's knee.

A nursing history sheet adapted for use with children is used. When the child is admitted in an emergency, only brief essential details are taken and the student will need guidance on what is essential information. If a parent is staying with the child, there is less pressure to elicit every detail, for the gaps can be filled in later. Many of the questions should be addressed to an older child as much as to his parents.

Recording the information

There are no rules about taking a nursing history or about asking questions in a specific order. Much information can be gained in a friendly conversation, when the nurse shows interest, and it reduces the cross-questioning effect.

Information which may be requested in the history sheet is set out here.

Personal details
Full name, first name and pet name, address
Age, date of birth, birth weight
Religion, baptised
Next of kin: relationship, address, telephone number
General practitioner, health visitor/clinic, school or play group.

Family
Child's name for parents
Siblings, names and ages
Pets with names
Mode of transport—own car, bus, public transport.

This admission
Reason for admission
Child's knowledge about his condition
Parents' knowledge about child's condition
Recent contact with infectious disease
Is the child taking any medicines?
How does the child take tablets?

Home routine
Diet
Baby—feeding routine, brand of milk, times, weaning diet
Child—likes and dislikes, favourite food and drink
Method—bottle, spoon, teacher beaker, knife and fork
Feeds self or needs help
Special diet for cultural, religious or medical reasons.
Elimination
Urinary—control, day and night
  Does child wear napkins?
  Special word to communicate need
  Toilet, pot, recently trained, needs help
  Any problems?
Bowels—any problems?
Sleep
Bed or cot, shares bed
Time of going to bed, sleeping pattern at night
Daytime rest, length and time of day
What helps child to settle.
Mobility
Average for age, i.e. sit, crawl, walk
Help needed with bathing, dressing.

Emotional aspects
Response to this admission
Favourite toy or cuddly
Any previous hospital admissions, reactions and how helped
Previous separations from mother or home
Any unusual situations at home, e.g. family problem, new baby.

Physical assessment
General appearance—normal, obese
Condition of skin—good, rashes, spots, bruises or broken areas, dehydrated, oedematous
Condition of hair—clean, dirty, infested
Speech—limitations, difficulty, language problem
Hearing
Sight   —normal, degree or disability, help needed.

Observations
Temperature, pulse rate, respirations, colour, pain, weight, height, urinalysis.

Comments on taking a history

The nursing history sheet contains many of these questions in order to remind the nurse about the information which is needed, and to reduce the amount of writing. The child's level of dependence and abilities need to be established at the outset so that staff can assess whether he is regressing developmentally. The effect of his illness on activities of living is also required. Family and social problems have a greater influence on children than on adults and a social history is usually recorded by the doctor, or by the social worker if there is a problem.

The nurse should be selective in the questions she asks, which should be relevant to the child's age and stage of development. The 5-year-old will not appreciate being asked if he needs help with feeding. Repetitive questioning on the same subject should be avoided, so if medical staff routinely record the same information, for example on the child's immunisations and the infectious diseases he has had, this can be taken from the medical records and the parents spared unnecessary questioning. Having completed the assessment, the nurse should have started to build up a relationship with the family, learning about the child's background, his problems, his strengths and some of the difficulties he may have.

Planning

Using the initial nursing assessment, the child's problems are identified. These problems are what the child or his parents see as problems and not what the nurse sees as problems. They may be described as actual or potential problems and writing (p) beside the latter saves time and avoids unnecessary writing. Having identified problems, goals or objectives can be set to solve or reduce them. Short-term, medium and long-term goals may be required for the same patient.

Karen (aged 14 months) is a good example (see p. 4). She is confined to her cot in a head-down position with her legs in traction. This normally cheerful little girl is fractious and reluctant to drink. A long-term goal of her medical and nursing care is that after completion of treatment and rehabilitation, her physical development will be normal for her age. This is unlikely to be achieved for many months.

A short-term problem

Karen's reluctance to drink is identified by the nurse as a short-term and high priority problem, and her mother agrees. They discuss various solutions sharing their expertise, the mother an expert on Karen and the nurse experienced in caring for young children on traction. Karen's mother thinks she would drink better from the beaker she uses at home and the staff nurse realises that Karen has not had time to adjust to the abnormal pull on her abdominal muscles, and might take frequent small drinks better than larger amounts less often. She might also benefit from analgesia to relieve the discomfort.

An objective is set, which is that Karen will take 500 ml of fluid in the next 24 hours. Karen's mother and the nurse discuss the action to be taken to achieve this and they formulate a plan. The problem is recorded in the nursing Kardex:

Problem	Objective	Nursing care	Evaluation
Refuses to drink	To drink 500 ml by 9 a.m. 6/3/87	1. Use own mug 2. Offer maximum 60 ml fluid hourly 3. Give Calpol 4 hrly if restless or fractious	6/3/87 9 a.m. objective achieved Increase intake to 600 ml by 7/3/87

Evaluation

Because the objective is measurable and timed, there will be no doubt about the outcome. After 24 hours the situation is evaluated by the nurse and Karen's mother. Assessment at this stage is based on whether the objective has been achieved. In fact Karen had taken 520 ml of fluid so it had been achieved. If the objective had been described as 'increase fluid intake' and the nursing plan had read 'push fluids', no-one would have known whether the objective had been achieved or not.

Evaluation also involves a decision on continuing the care as planned, modifying it, trying a different method or if Karen was drinking well considering the problem solved and cancelling it in the nursing record. In the latter case it might remain as a potential problem. As 500 ml of fluid was less than the recommended fluid intake for her weight, and because she was drinking more willingly, the target figure was raised to 600 ml for the next 24 hours.

Karen had other problems during the first few days. These included discomfort due to her position, frustration at not being able to move, refusing to eat unless she could feed herself, soreness of skin due to pressure (p), not being cuddled and touched as much as usual, constipation (p) and not being able to play normally.

Children adapt amazingly quickly to new situations and within a few days Karen was much more settled, some of her problems had been resolved and she was tolerating her restricted existence more happily.

REFERENCES AND FURTHER READING

Organisation of care
Consumers' Association 1980 Children in hospital. A 'Which' Investigation. Consumers' Association, London
Meadows R 1969 The captive mother. Archives of Disease in Childhood 44 (235)

Planning care
Orem D E 1971 Nursing: concepts of practice. McGraw-Hill, New York
Roper N, Logan W W, Tierney A J 1985 The elements of nursing, 2nd edn. Churchill Livingstone, Edinburgh

PART | TWO

The child's
background

The child's background

Parents' roles in child
    rearing
Day care of pre-school
    children
    Childminder
    Day nursery
    Nursery school
    Playgroup

Disadvantaged children
Influences on family life
Prenatal influences on
    the child
    Genetics
    Factors affecting fetal
        development

4

The family

The majority of children today are brought up in a family setting. From time to time, the family as a social group is threatened by external pressures in society but so far it has adapted and survived as a social institution in which the young are nurtured and protected during a long period of dependence. A home where there is loving care in a secure setting, freedom to develop and explore the world, stimulation to learn and a guiding hand, gives the child the best possible foundation for life.

Provision of this type of home is not dependent on one 'best buy' pattern of family living, nor is it dependent on wealth. Families where father goes out to work and mother stays at home caring for the children may be considered by most people as the norm, but there are numerous other ways of organising the family which many parents choose or circumstances dictate.

PARENTS' ROLES IN CHILD REARING

1. With two parents

a. Father works, mother stays at home and cares for the children

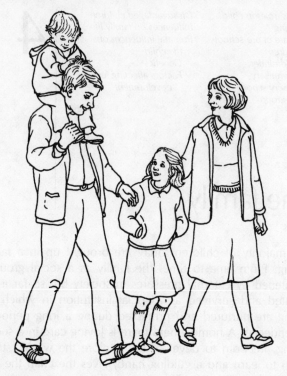

Fig. 4.1 Family setting of two parents.

b. Father works full-time and takes over the care of the children while his wife works part-time, probably working an evening or night shift.
c. Mother and father reverse roles. Mother goes to work, father does the housework and cares for the children.

   Both parents may prefer this arrangement, the mother may want to continue her career full-time, her salary may be more than her husband's, or he may be unemployed.
d. Father and mother both work full-time and delegate the day care of the children to other people.
e. Both parents may be unemployed. They may share the children's care.

2. One parent family (OPF)

The single parent may be unmarried, separated or divorced, widow or widower. Of all OPFs, 38% are headed by a divorced mother (1983) compared with 27% in 1975. Some women decide to have a child and remain single, others may become foster mothers.

OPFs are often at a disadvantage when compared with other families. They are more likely to have financial problems, but other factors such as loneliness and lack of support can also make life difficult for these parents.

3. Group care

a. A few children live in small communities such as communes or the kibbutzim of Israel. Although this is unusual in the UK, it is quite common in other parts of the world.
b. Children's homes
   Approximately 34 000 children live in residential homes. They are in the care of the local authority and may be there temporarily, or permanently until they are 18 years old. In some instances the parents may have asked for the child to be taken into care during a family crisis (voluntary care). Other children are taken into care compulsorily either because their home is unsuitable or because they are out of control. Many of the children in long-term care are found foster homes.

For centuries most members of the family lived, worked and died in the same locality. They were therefore available to support and help each other. The young mother would rely on her own mother for advice about the new baby and unmarried aunts and grandparents would 'mind' the children.

Smaller families and increasing mobility

Many young mothers today live too far away from their parents for them to provide close support, possibly living in a

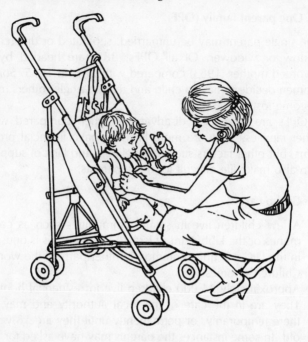

Fig 4.2 Isolation can be a problem for some mothers.

strange town without friends or familiar neighbours. The less fortunate may be living in a high rise block of flats, and be isolated all day with no company and no-one at hand to turn to if help is needed.

Smaller families and the increasing mobility of the population result in more mothers with young children being isolated in this way.

Working mothers

As a result of the changing role of women in society and equal opportunities for women, many married women have the choice of continuing to work full-time or of remaining at home and looking after the children. Making the decision can be stressful for women who are torn between continuing a satisfying career and being with the children during their formative years. Some postpone returning to work until the children start school or later.

Factors which the woman has to take into consideration include her husband's views and willingness to help, the stress of doing two jobs, the effect on the children, suitable arrangements for the care of the children and contingency plans in case they are ill. The working mother may have feelings of guilt about neglecting the children or feel more fulfilled because she is working.

DAY CARE OF PRE-SCHOOL CHILDREN

There are several alternative types of care for young children whose parents are unable to look after them during the day. Many families with a fit grandmother living within easy travelling distance, depend on her to look after the children, if she is able and willing to do so. Of course some grandmothers now work as well and are therefore unable to oblige, although most enjoy the involvement. The advantage for the child is that he is with a familiar adult and for the parents that it is free. A disadvantage is that the child may not receive the stimulation he needs from an older person. If this is a problem the child can attend a playgroup or day nursery for part of the day.

Childminder

A childminder looks after a small group of children in her own home and provides for all their needs for part or all of the day. The children must be less than 5 years old and unrelated to the childminder, who must be approved and registered with the local authority. In spite of the regulations many women who are not registered take children into their homes, and these are often the ones who are least concerned about providing a suitable environment for the children. The parents pay a mutually agreed fee for child-minding.

Day nursery

The day nursery caters for children from the age of 6 months to 5 years and is usually open from 8 a.m. until 6 p.m. The hours of attendance are arranged for the individual child and this may be a temporary measure for a few weeks or a permanent arrangement. A child whose mother is in hospital might attend each afternoon for 2 weeks; another child may attend every day on a regular basis because his unmarried mother has a full-time job. Children from homes where there are problems such as a single parent family are given priority when children are selected for nurseries.

The children are divided into small family groups with a regular member of staff who is usually a trained nursery nurse. Children therefore have a familiar caretaker to whom they can relate. A good nursery provides a stimulating environment and encourages parents to join in activities with their children if they wish.

Some places are allotted to children from disadvantaged homes and special help may be given to these children and their parents. Most nurseries also give priority to handicapped children so that the child can benefit from the stimulating environment. It provides an opportunity for him to mix with other children and to become less dependent on his parents. It also gives the parents a break from looking after him.

Nursery school

This is a mixture of nursery and school as the name suggests. It is administered as part of the school system and therefore has the same hours and holidays. This makes nursery schools of limited value to working parents. The children, aged 3 to

5 years, are divided into classes, each with its own qualified teacher and team of nursery nurses.

The function of the nursery school is not to teach reading, writing and arithmetic, but to provide a stimulating environment which will help the young child's development. Free activity, stimulating play, the use of educational toys, and informal group activities such as musical games which help social development, are all part of the nursery school day. There are always some children with special needs who have been given a place because of their unsatisfactory background or unstimulating environment at home. They receive extra help for specific problems, perhaps retarded speech and language development or an inability to mix with other children.

Nursery classes are attached to infant schools in some areas, run on the same lines as nursery schools. The transition to school at 5 years is made easier for these children because the nursery classes are normally housed in the school building and they may share some of the facilities. Some infant schools take children who have reached their fourth birthday.

Playgroup

Playgroups may be run by groups of mothers, privately by qualified people such as nursery nurses or by charities such as Save the Children Fund or the NSPCC. The local authority is responsible for maintaining the standard of premises, staffing and equipment which is laid down by law. It does this by inspections, giving approval and maintaining a register of playgroups. Children are mostly between 3 and 5 years old.

There is no set structure for playgroups but parents are usually closely involved and a fee is charged. Most playgroups receive financial help from the local authority, and social service departments may pay the fees for children from needy families.

Other types of day care

Creches are set up by businesses, universities or hospitals on the work site to provide care for employees' or students' children. Creches are conveniently close at hand for parents taking and collecting their children, and the parent is available in an emergency. The standard of care depends on those running it, who do not need to be qualified.

DISADVANTAGED CHILDREN

The vast majority of parents rear their children without any special help by using their common sense, and taking advice from relatives, friends and members of the community health team.

A minority of families cannot cope, either because of the magnitude of their problems or because of their limitations, and children from these families are the deprived ones whose development is likely to be slow. Statistics also show that they are more likely to become ill, to be admitted to hospital and to have a fatal illness than the average child. 20% of children in paediatric wards in the UK have a disorder totally or partly related to social problems (see Ch. 12).

INFLUENCES ON FAMILY LIFE

Culture

The population of the UK includes many different ethnic groups. Immigrants from the Indian subcontinent range from those who are educated, articulate and hardworking, among them many professional people, to those who are poor, socially isolated and vulnerable. The women in the latter group often have most difficulty when their child is ill. Communication is difficult when the mother does not speak

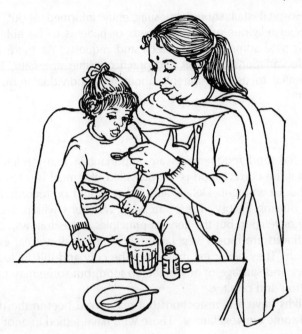

Fig 4.3 Supplementing the diet with vitamins.

English. Sometimes the other children act as interpreters or the husband, who is usually with his wife, may speak for her.

In every society, strongly held beliefs and customs about child rearing are common. Infant feeding and weaning may cause problems. For example a child may be given only milk for the first 2 years of life, after which he may be weaned on rice and puréed fruit, which results in nutritional deficiency.

Asian children are more likely to develop rickets than their British friends because of their diet, for the flour and fat used in cooking are not fortified with vitamins as the British equivalents are. Another reason is lack of sunshine to their skin, due to their clothing covering most of the body, and the habit of staying indoors.

Hospital staff should be sufficiently informed about the special religious or cultural needs of patients to be able to anticipate some of their needs and requests. As there are wide variations of belief and practice within any faith, it is essential to ask the parents about their individual requirements.

Diet

Special food requirements are important in many religions and if the correct food is not provided, the meal is often left without comment. Details about diet should be recorded in the nursing history. There are wide variations within a culture or religion but the general principles are as follows.

Hindus are mostly vegetarian and some may not eat eggs or fish. They never eat meat from the cow and this includes gravy and sausage or any made up food, but some may take mutton and poultry.

Sikhs have few restrictions but may avoid beef in the diet and some are vegetarians. Those who have settled in another country are usually very liberal.

Muslims abstain from eating pork or any food which contains pork products. Their meat has to be ritually slaughtered and is called halal meat. Most Muslims accept Kosher meat.

Jews do not eat pork or pork products.

Providing permitted foods does not guarantee that children or adults will eat it, for British food often seems strange and tasteless to them. Ideally the meal should be food suited to their taste which they can enjoy.

Attitudes and customs

Other differences in attitudes and customs which may emerge when a child is in hospital with his mother are likely to relate to hygiene, acceptance of drugs, certain treatments or attitudes towards the handicapped.

Politics

Government departments concerned with health, welfare and education are all closely involved with child care. Child allowances, the school-leaving age and regulations about playgroups are examples of aspects of children's lives controlled by central government. Government policies are embodied in new laws, for example the Family Law (Scotland) 1985 and the 1982 Education Act (England and Wales). The government also sets up committees to review a specific service or situation and to recommend any changes necessary. The Court Report (1976) on child health services in Britain which took 3 years to complete is a good example. Statutory inquiries may be set up in cases of child abuse to investigate the incident and to recommend any changes in management which would help to prevent a recurrence.

Local councils are also responsible for allocating public funds. Will they spend money on refurbishing the town hall or on creating a play area for children who have to play in the street?

Medical and technological advances

Increasing knowledge in fields such as child development, genetics, pharmacology and immunology have contributed to improved standards of health and more effective treatment of sick children. Less invasive techniques in diagnostic procedures, more sophisticated laboratory tests and some advances in the care of pre-term babies as well as in intensive care of children have been due to advances in technology.

Changes in society

The standard of living for most families has risen steadily since the Second World War. Greater affluence is apparent in the consumption of more expensive foods though not necessarily a healthier diet, more people owning their house, more holidays and travel abroad. Around 50% of households have a deep freeze or a fridge-freezer, 74% have a colour television and an increasing number have video recorders and computers.

More money is spent on children's toys and clothes, on presents and expensive leisure activities. There are many more opportunities for young people to participate in outdoor pursuits and special interest holidays which encourage the development of self-reliance and confidence. A few of these opportunities are available for the less well off but most are for those who can afford to pay. At the other end of the scale 14% of the population are either unemployed, poorly paid or single parents with an inadequate income.

Discipline

Children in general appear to be less disciplined than previously. This is evident in schools but may well stem from the early years at home. Over the last 30 years more emphasis has been placed on allowing the child freedom to develop his potential and this has been interpreted literally by some parents who do not discipline their children at all. Without any control when they are younger, children have nothing on which to build self-control later on. Many children are left to fend for themselves while their parents are engrossed in their social life or out at work, and are more likely to have problems. Lacking attention and left to their own devices, they soon find themselves in trouble.

The permissive society

The relaxation of long-established codes of behaviour relating to marriage and sexual relationships has resulted in what many people call the permissive society. Abortion, illegitimacy, divorce, homosexuality and unmarried couples living together have all become more accepted. While a more liberal atmosphere may be beneficial to adults in some situations, the children are the ones who are the most likely to suffer as a result. During 1984 divorce affected 149 000 children in the UK. The atmosphere in the home before the divorce and the adjustments which children are required to make afterwards can be devastating. Krementz (1985) interviewed children of parents who said that their divorce had been easy, and found that their children did not agree. She found that children talking about their parents' divorce were more unhappy than others whose parent had died.

Alcohol, drugs and promiscuity

Adolescents have more choices and freedom to decide how they will spend their time and their money than previously. Parents have correspondingly more anxiety about their children at this age. Alcohol consumption among young people has doubled since 1950 and cheaper drugs which are more easily obtained have contributed to a rapid increase in the number of people taking drugs. The number of illegitimate births continues to rise (110 000 in 1984), and promiscuity in adolescents is implicated in the rising incidence of carcinoma of the cervix in young women, which rarely occurred previously. Alcohol, drugs and promiscuity are not only immediate problems but have long-term, irreversible effects.

Television

Television is a mixed blessing. Children can learn much about a variety of topics related to the arts, science and the world around them. However, watching television encourages the child to be a passive observer which may become a habit extending beyond the television screen. The many addicts who spend more time watching television than they do at school, miss out on creative activities, social interaction, and other experiences which are a valuable part of development.

Violence on television is suspected of influencing viewers' attitudes and in some cases behaviour. Young children are likely to accept people on television as models while older children are more likely to experiment by copying actions which may be undesirable or dangerous.

A less obvious influence of television is the portrayal of family life. The unrealistic and glamourous lifestyles of TV fiction easily become models which influence the unwitting viewers' expectations of their own family life. However in programmes portraying more realistic families, the dramatic moments are quite likely to be concerned with bedroom scenes, drug-taking or a pregnant teenager and could perhaps be translated to real life more easily than the glamorous life.

Advertisements, too, encourage false assumptions. Using a certain brand of soap powder or disinfectant is associated with being a good mother. The perfect baby in spotless clothes, taking his weaning diet without spilling a drop, is not true to life but inexperienced mothers do not know this and so pick up unrealistic expectations about their baby's abilities.

PRENATAL INFLUENCES ON THE CHILD

Genetics

Differences in human beings are the result of each individual's genetic inheritance and the environment in which he has developed and lived. The relative importance of nature (genetic make-up) and nurture (the developing child's environment) has always been a favourite topic for discussion. Many people now agree that heredity determines the maximum level of achievement (the potential), while the environment affects to what extent this will be achieved. For example, the newborn baby who has inherited from his father the potential to play the violin brilliantly, suffers brain damage at birth which causes spasticity. As a result he is never able to develop his musical talent. The environment

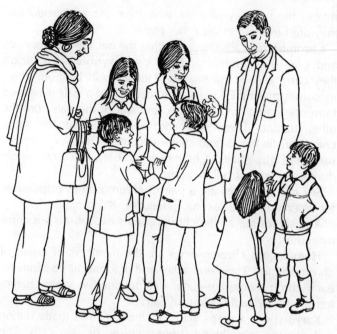

Fig. 4.4 Genetic inheritance determines individual characteristics.

before and during delivery is as important as at any time thereafter.

Genetic disease has become relatively more important in child care in the Western world because other conditions which previously caused ill health and death have been conquered. About one-quarter of all deaths in the first year of life is due to congenital abnormalities. A number of these will be due to a genetic disorder.

Definitions

These definitions are given as a brief introduction for students who have not studied the subject previously and to refresh the memory of those who have. As an introduction they are best read in the order given.

Chromosomes are situated within the nucleus of every cell and consist of protein and DNA (deoxyribonucleic acid); they carry genetic information. Human cells have 46 chromosomes making 23 pairs, one member of a pair is derived from one parent and the other member of the pair from the other parent. These two chromosomes have the same characteristic length and shape except for the sex chromosomes in the male. Chromosomes only become visible during the time of cell division.

Sex chromosomes are a pair of chromosomes responsible for determining the sex: XX in females, XY in males.

Autosomes are all the chromosomes except the sex chromosomes.

Homologous chromosomes are the members of a pair of chromosomes. They look alike, and at identical positions on each chromosome are genes determining the same characteristic, for example colour of hair.

Karyotype is a preparation of chromosomes made during cell division from blood, bone marrow or skin cells. The

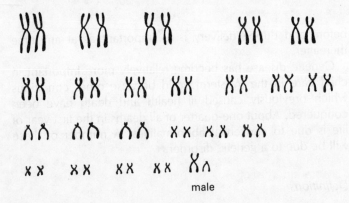

male

Fig. 4.5 The karyotype of a normal human male. The chromosomes are numbered and grouped according to size and shape.

chromosomes are numbered and grouped according to size and shape (Fig. 4.5). Fetal skin cells from amniotic fluid can be karyotyped and used to diagnose some abnormalities before birth.

Genes are the units of inheritance occupying a specific site (locus) on a chromosome. They consist of part of the DNA molecule and are paired as the chromosomes are. That means on the same site of each of the chromosomes of one pair there is a gene for the same trait.

Allele is a matching but not identical gene, which means it is in the same position on the corresponding chromosome, as in the person who has a gene for black hair on one of the chromosomes and a gene for blond hair on the other chromosome.

Genotype is the genetic constitution of an individual.

Phenotype is the physical appearance, the biochemical and physiological make-up of an individual which is the result of the genotype plus environmental factors.

Homozygous means having identical genes at a gene locus on each of a pair of homologous chromosomes, for instance both genes being for black hair.

Heterozygous means having alleles at a gene locus on each of a pair of homologous chromosomes, as in the example given for allele.

Abnormalities

Mosaic describes an individual who has some abnormal cells. For example an individual may be a mosaic of normal and trisomy 21 cells. This means that some of his cells have two No. 21 chromosomes (as normal) but other cells have three No. 21 chromosomes. Trisomy 21 leads to Down's syndrome.

Mutation describes a change in gene or chromosome structure during early development so that the resulting individual has new characteristics. Not all mutations produce disorder and some may be beneficial.

Patterns of inheritance

Dominant when related to patterns of inheritance means that one abnormal gene causes the disease.

Recessive means that the disease is caused by two abnormal genes, one from each parent.

Autosomal dominant inheritance. The abnormal gene is carried on one of a pair of autosomes. Because it is dominant, those with just one abnormal gene are affected by the disease. Where one of the parents carries the gene, the chance of their children having the disease is 50:50.

Autosomal recessive inheritance. The parents, who must each have one abnormal gene, are asymptomatic. Their children have a 1 in 4 chance of having the disease by inheriting one gene from each parent. Tests are available which detect carriers of some recessively inherited diseases.

Sex linked recessive inheritance. The small Y chromosome in the male carries only information relating to gender. The recessive gene on the male's X chromosome is therefore unopposed and all males with this gene are affected. The female with the abnormal gene is a carrier because only one of her two X chromosomes has the recessive gene. The chance of her sons having the disease is 50:50; there is the same chance of her daughters being carriers.

Multifactorial inheritance. It is quite common to have an unusually high incidence of a disorder in a family without any identifiable pattern of inheritance. Environmental factors are known to be relevant in some cases and probably play an important role in many disorders. A genetic predisposition to a disorder combined with specific environmental conditions results in the occurrence of the disease. The cause is therefore partly genetic, partly environmental, hence its name. Examples of this type of disorder are cleft lip and palate, pyloric stenosis in infancy and spina bifida.

Genetic counselling

Couples may seek help from a genetic counsellor before

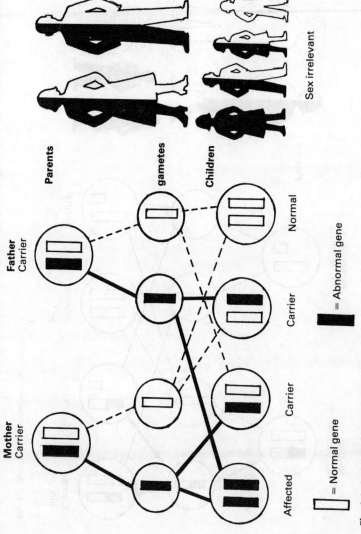

Fig. 4.6 Autosomal recessive inheritance.

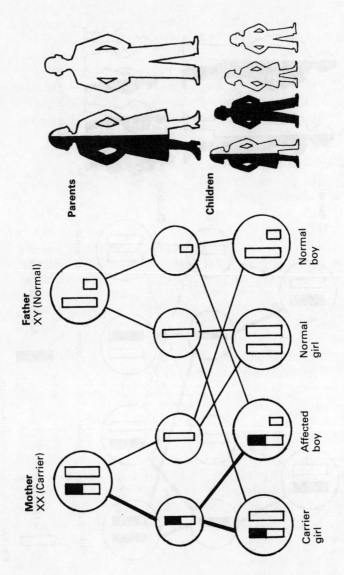

Fig 4.7 Sex-linked recessive inheritance.

marriage if they have a family history of inherited disease or if they are related to each other. With modern screening procedures some couples learn that their unborn child has an inherited disorder; many other parents see a genetic counsellor for the first time after the birth of an affected child.

When an inherited disease has been diagnosed, details of the child's background are recorded including the obstetric history. A family tree is compiled going back three generations in order to identify family members who suffered from the same condition. If there is a clearly defined pattern of inheritance in the family or the genetic cause of the child's disorder is known, the risk of siblings being affected can be calculated accurately.

Parents are advised about the risk of future children being affected. If an exact figure cannot be given, it may be possible to give some indication of the probability. The parents are given information about the disease, its effect and treatment. They may be referred to family planning clinics, and to other agencies for further help, if they wish. When the disorder is diagnosed in pregnancy, parents are informed about the implications for them and for the child, and the options open to them are explained. Counselling and support are provided before and after the parents decide whether they wish to have the baby or to terminate the pregnancy.

Factors affecting fetal development

The first 8 weeks of the embryo's development is rapid, complex and fascinating. By the time it is 4 cm long, at 10 weeks, all its basic systems are formed. Although the fetus is well protected from most environmental dangers, certain factors, transmitted through the mother, are known to be potentially harmful.

1. Viral infections may affect the development of vital organs. Rubella is a well-known example which is likely to

result in fetal death or the baby having congenital defects such as cataract, a heart defect or deafness. Auto-immune deficiency syndrome (AIDS) is caused by a new virus human immunodeficiency virus (HIV) that can affect the newborn infant. Vaccines may be equally dangerous and should not be given to pregnant women.

2. Radiation before 28 weeks of pregnancy has, in a few cases, been associated with developmental abnormalities or leukaemia in the child.

3. Some chemicals and drugs, including non-prescribed ones, may affect fetal development, so the pregnant woman is advised to take as little medication as possible. Her doctor advises on continuing any regular medication which she has been prescribed.

4. Smoking. Babies of mothers who smoke, weigh less at birth than those of non-smokers and are therefore prone to more problems in the neonatal period. The mortality rate is also higher for small babies.

5. Drug addiction in the mother can result in the newborn baby being dependent on the drug. Excessive alcohol consumption may cause deformities in the fetus.

REFERENCES AND FURTHER READING

Social background
Bewley B 1986 The epidemiology of adolescent behaviour problems. British Medical Bulletin 42 (2): 200–203
Central Statistical Office 1986 Social Trends 16. HMSO, London
Doust M 1983 Family breakdown. Nursing 2 (20): 584–585
General Nursing Council 1982 Aspects of sick children's nursing: a learning package. GNC for England and Wales (now English National Board), London. Study Unit 8 Cultural differences
Krementz J 1986 How it feels when parents divorce. Gollancz, London
Lobo E D H 1978 Children of immigrant families to Britain. Hodder & Stoughton, London
Macfarlane J A 1984 Progress in child health. Churchill Livingstone, Edinburgh, ch 10 Children and divorce

Genetics
Fitzsimmons J S, Fitzsimmons E M 1980 Handbook of clinical genetics. Heinemann, London

Principles and trends
The first year
1–2 years
2–4 years
4–7 years
7–12 years
Adolescence

5

Development

PRINCIPLES AND TRENDS

Growth is visible and therefore comes to mind first when development is mentioned. However psychological (emotional), intellectual (mental or cognitive), social and spiritual aspects are equally, if not more, important. All aspects of development are really inseparable but they provide convenient sub-divisions when studying the subject, as long as it is always borne in mind that each one affects every other one.

Milestones

Development progresses in steps and stages, sometimes marked by a single action or achievement as when a baby smiles for the first time or first stands alone. The delight on the parents' face and their excited response at each new achievement is exactly what the baby needs to encourage him in his progress to the next stage. These milestones of development are often used to assess the child's progress in the early years. Physically or mentally handicapped children are likely to be retarded in some aspects of development but rarely all, and therefore each child needs to be assessed individually, for slowness in one area does not necessarily mean slowness in another.

Stages and ages

There is a wide age range within which normal children attain any particular level of development. For example, the average age for standing alone is 13 months, but a child who is developing normally may reach this stage any time from 9 to 14 months or even later. However the average age of attainment is useful as a rough guide. Parents often need reassurance that their young child is not backward because, for example, he may be slower to talk than his older sisters were at the same age. Each child goes at his own pace and all children pass through the same stages in the same sequence. Each stage is affected by those preceding it and influences those following. Environmental factors may affect the rate of development as in the 10-month-old baby who was unable to sit up unsupported. His mother had been very withdrawn due to undiagnosed postnatal depression, and had nursed him lying flat on her knee for several months. In contrast, African babies who are carried on their mothers' backs from birth, are able to sit up earlier than British babies.

Patterns of development

The orderly and logical sequence of development in all its aspects is fascinating and is exemplified in two directional trends in the infant's growth and attainment of motor skills which are dependent on the maturation of the nervous system.

a. The child develops from head-to-tail or cephalocaudally. The newborn baby's head (and brain) is large when compared with his legs, but this is to the baby's advantage for his nervous system is sufficiently developed to co-

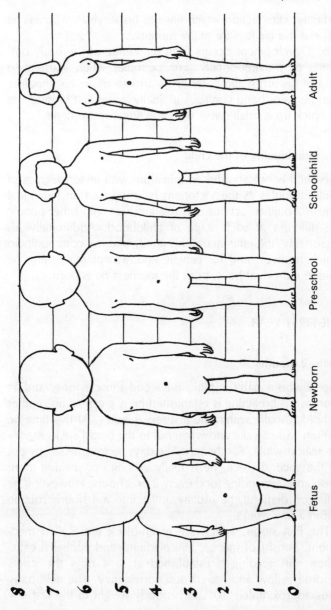

Fig. 5.1 Changing proportions of the human body

ordinate reflex action which ensures his survival, whereas he will not use his legs for many months.

b. Development occurs from the centre of the body outwards or proximodistally. For example, when learning to control his arms, the baby first learns to move his shoulder then he gains hand control and finally by his first birthday he can pick up a small sweet with fine finger movements.

The individuality of the child

The child is not an adult in miniature with lesser degrees of adult attributes as the Victorians believed, but an individual whose thoughts, actions and relationships with other people are different at each stage of childhood. Additionally his personality, the influence of his family and the community in which he lives, and his genetic endowment make him the unique individual he is, from the moment he is born.

THE FIRST YEAR

Birth–2 months

The newborn baby is pink, has good muscle tone, and as soon as his breathing is established he is given to his mother to hold, usually within the first few minutes. At this time he is often wide awake and when put to the breast sucks readily for a short while. For the next few days he may be sleepy but by the second week, he is really waking up, making more noise and demanding food every 2 or 3 hours. However if he is fed on demand, he usually settles into a 4 hourly routine within a few weeks.

The first stools, which are green-black and called meconium, consist of mucus, bile pigments and epithelial cells. When milk feeding is established at 3–4 days the stools become yellow and have a soft consistency. The new baby loses approximately 10% of his body weight in the first few

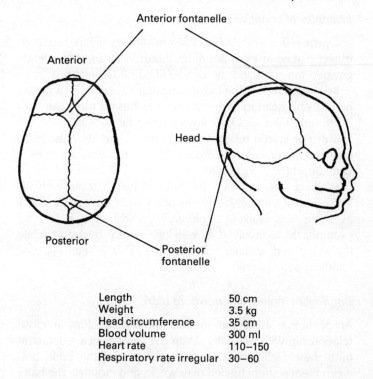

Length	50 cm
Weight	3.5 kg
Head circumference	35 cm
Blood volume	300 ml
Heart rate	110–150
Respiratory rate irregular	30–60

Fig. 5.2 The newborn baby. The posterior and anterior fontanelles close by 8 weeks and 18 months respectively: these so-called 'soft spots' are not delicate as many mothers think.

days, but should regain this by the tenth day. Many babies develop physiological jaundice in the first week of life which disappears by the second week and rarely requires any treatment.

The newborn baby's movements are haphazard or reflex and he has no head control. He can suck, swallow, vomit, cough and yawn; he turns away from a bright light and is startled by a loud noise. He also has primitive reflexes which are present at birth but disappear in the first year.

Examples of primitive reflexes

Grasp reflex. The baby closes his fingers tightly round an object placed in the palm of his hand. With an adult's finger grasped in each hand, he can be lifted off the mattress.

Rooting reflex. If the baby's cheek is stroked with a finger, he turns his head to that side and searches for the finger with his mouth, then sucks vigorously when he finds it.

Moro or startle reflex. In reaction to a sudden noise or to his head being suddenly dropped back, his arms are thrown wide apart then close over his chest.

Walking reflex. When the baby is held upright with his feet on a flat surface, he moves one foot in front of the other as if he was walking. Voluntary control of muscles, for example those involved in walking, cannot be learnt while the associated walking reflex persists. This is seen in some handicapped children.

Bonding of mother and newborn baby

At or before birth the mother usually develops a close relationship with her baby. With the first physical contact at birth these feelings are often intensified and the bond between them is strengthened over weeks and months. The baby responds to her loving touch, and emotional and physical satisfaction are simultaneous and mutual. Bonding is disrupted if the mother and baby are separated, in which case it may be difficult to re-establish the relationship. Whenever possible mother and baby should be kept together, and if the baby needs specialised care in another hospital, the mother should be transferred with him. There is some evidence that separation of mother and baby in the neonatal period may result in a greater risk of child abuse subsequently.

Continuing development of mother and baby attachment

During the early months, the baby grows accustomed to his mother's handling. He is not aware of her as a separate

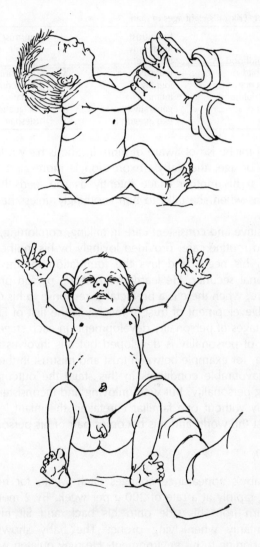

Fig. 5.3 Head lag and the Moro response at 1 month.

Table 5.1 Erikson's eight ages of man

Infancy	basic trust	v.	mistrust
Toddler	autonomy	v.	shame, doubt
Early childhood	initiative	v.	guilt
Schoolchild	industry	v.	inferiority
Adolescence	identity	v.	role confusion
Young adulthood	intimacy	v.	isolation
Adulthood	generativity	v.	stagnation
Maturity	ego integrity	v.	despair

person for he is not aware of himself. She is his world. By 4 weeks of age, the baby's expression is more alert and he stares at his mother's face intently as she feeds him. He quietens when she talks to him soothingly unless he is very hungry.

Sensitive and consistent care in talking, comforting, touching and routine care, provided lovingly by his mother, satisfies all his needs and lays the foundation for the baby's emotional security. He learns to trust the person providing the care, when there is a predictable response to his cries for help. Development of trust in infancy is the first of Erikson's eight stages of personality development. In each stage, some aspect of personality is developed but this involves internal conflict, for example between trust and mistrust in the infant. With favourable conditions in this stage the outcome is a trusting personality, but with unloving and inconsistent care, possibly without one familiar caretaker, the infant learns to mistrust the world and this becomes part of his personality.

Growth

The baby's appearance changes each week, for he gains weight rapidly at a rate of 200 g per week. By 2 months he can turn from his side onto his back and lift his head momentarily when lying prone. The baby shows signs of responding to his environment. He may quieten when he is picked up or may lie awake staring around. When he is hungry or uncomfortable he cries lustily and reacts with generalised movements of his whole body.

First smile

Around 6 weeks of age the baby smiles for the first time. Fleeting smiles before this are often due to wind but there is no doubt about the first true smile. As well as smiling, the baby's eyes light up, usually in response to a familiar face. This first social contact with another person is a landmark in human development. By 8 weeks the baby is making cooing and gurgling noises, and his mother can differentiate between his cries of hunger, boredom and discomfort.

3–5 months

The 3-month-old baby is awake for longer periods during the day but may still require 4 hourly feeds day and night. He can hold a rattle placed in his hand although he has little control over it and lacks the hand-eye co-ordination to look at it at the same time. Through playing with his fingers and at the same time watching, feeling sensation and movement in them, he gradually learns that they are part of himself.

Responding to his environment

The baby is contented and responds happily to other people, particularly his mother and other family members whose voices he recognises. He smiles and gurgles when spoken to and will lie in his cot 'talking' to himself. He listens to people talking and will turn his head in response to a voice.

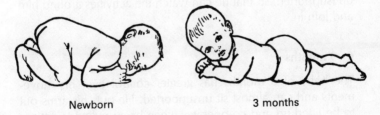

Newborn   3 months

Fig. 5.4 The newborn baby and at 3 months.

He makes excited noises and kicks his legs at the sight of his feeding bottle. He is at his most sociable and encourages everyone to pay attention to him. He accepts strangers happily and shows annoyance if they ignore him.

Everything to his mouth

The baby starts to reach for and grasp toys and from 4 months everything goes to his mouth. Through this hand/mouth approach the baby learns about his environment. He explores anything within reach; fingers, toes and clothes are conveniently close and never fall out of reach. Freud called this the oral stage of development in which the child gains pleasure from oral sensations such as sucking, licking and chewing.

Weaning

Weaning from milk to mixed diet is begun when the baby is about 4 months old and continues for several months. The 5-month-old starts to chew so this is a good time to introduce foods like rusks or large pieces of apple for the baby to chew. The first teeth may appear at this time but are not essential for chewing.

At 5 months the baby's weight is double his birth weight. He now benefits from being placed in different positions to encourage movement, for he is able to roll over onto his back from prone. He holds his head steady and prefers to sit up (supported) so that he can watch the activities around him and join in.

6–9 months

The baby of 6 months has greater control over his movements and can almost sit unsupported. He puts his arms out to be lifted up and co-operates when being pulled to sitting. He also enjoys bouncing up and down on an adult's knee, more so if it is accompanied by a rhyme or song. He is now able to pass a toy from one hand to the other.

By 9 months the baby sits unsupported and, if he is sitting on a firm surface, is sufficiently steady to be able to lean forward and pick up a toy. A few children start to crawl at this stage and to walk round the furniture holding on.

Psychosocial developments

At 6 months the child becomes increasingly interested in activities around him. He now has definite likes and dislikes and shouts to attract attention. He may laugh aloud with delight, or scream with anger and may also stiffen to resist being picked up. He babbles a variety of unintelligable sounds which have melody and variations in length.

Shy with strangers

Around 7 months of age the baby develops a shyness with strangers which develops into definite anxiety and dislike of unfamiliar people. This is due to the baby's newly acquired ability to distinguish between familiar and strange faces.

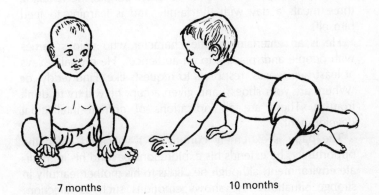

7 months   10 months

Fig. 5.5 The baby at 7 and 10 months.

Strangers therefore become a threat and the baby's attachment to his mother becomes stronger. He wants to be with his mother and will look around for her anxiously if she leaves the room.

10–12 months

The key word at this age is definitely 'mobility' though not necessarily on two feet. The baby starts to crawl in one of a variety of ways. He will either crawl on his hands and knees, shuffle forwards or backwards on his buttocks or move like a bear on all fours. Soon he is crawling with great skill at an incredible speed. By their first birthday, most children can walk with one hand held. The baby is able to pick up small objects neatly with thumb and tip of index finger in apposition (pincer grasp) and enjoys using this new skill.

Achievements at 1 year

The 1-year-old's achievements seem almost incredible when compared to the helpless newborn baby of the previous year. Not only is he mobile and almost on his feet, he has learnt to recognise and relate to other people, he is taking three meals a day with the family and is learning to feed himself.

He is an entertaining little character who enjoys games with people and 'playing to an audience'. He probably says at least two words, responds to requests like 'Find teddy' or 'Where are your shoes?' and given a cup, he will try to drink from it. These are all indications of normal intellectual development.

The baby is extremely curious at 1 year and given the opportunity, he extends his explorations beyond his immediate environment, although he clings to his mother fearfully in strange situations. He shows emotions such as affection, jealousy and anger, and although he manages to tolerate short delays in getting what he wants, he soon becomes

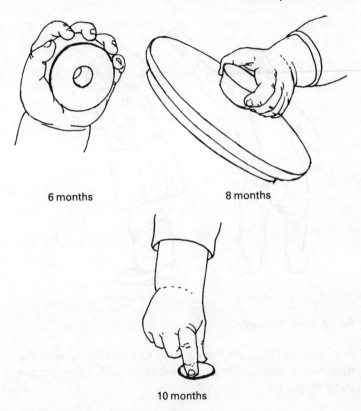

6 months

8 months

10 months

Fig. 5.6 The development of the pincer grasp.

frustrated. With a growing awareness of himself and his effect on those around him, he is quick to learn ways of gaining extra attention, for example after he has been tucked up in his cot for the night.

1–2 YEARS

The child's growth slows down in the 2nd year but nevertheless this is an exciting time for parents. The child takes his

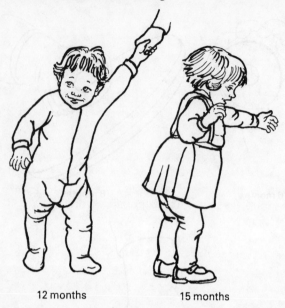

12 months   15 months

Fig. 5.7 1 year–15 months.

first steps and changes from a baby to a small child with the uniquely human ability to communicate with other people using language.

Walking unaided

By 15 months of age most children walk unaided though not necessarily steadily. The child's mother has to re-organise the house and put precious or dangerous objects out of reach for he has no sense of danger and always seems attracted to the least suitable objects such as glass ornaments.

The 1-year-old spends most of his time on the move, using his body, improving control of large muscles in walking, falling and rolling, learning to balance and co-ordinate his body. By his second birthday he can run, climb on furniture and negotiate stairs (holding the rail).

Learning to talk

This is another major achievement of the second year. From his first birthday he starts to say recognisable words, starting off with single ones. They serve as labels which may denote many aspects of the word. 'Teddy' may refer to the object but may also mean 'Teddy gone', or 'want Teddy'. One name also denotes many classes, for example 'dog' serves for cow, cat and horse. As vocabulary and understanding increase, the child progresses to a telegrammatic style of two- to three-word sentences. 'Drink Mummy' and 'No bed' are brief and to the point! The 2-year-old refers to himself by name and uses at least 50 recognisable words.

Dependence on mother

The child's attachment to his mother continues throughout the 2nd year to a greater or lesser degree, and reaches a peak around his second birthday. He is sometimes clinging and possessive towards her and tends to be jealous of any person or activity which comes between them.

Simon

While Simon's mother was enjoying talking to a friend over a cup of coffee, Simon, aged 20 months, was playing with his small cars on the floor nearby. He would normally do this quite happily as long as his mother was within sight or sound. Just when the conversation was most absorbing, Simon started to tease the dog and pull its tail. Simon's mother was forced to break off the conversation in order to rescue the dog and Simon received the attention he desired.

The child's comforter or 'cuddly' is never far away at this age. It is usually an old teddy or a ragged piece of material which was originally a blanket or a soft napkin placed under his head in his cot. It is indispensable when the child is distressed or tired and is often associated with going to sleep, so that the child may be unable to settle without it.

Sociability and play

Between 1 and 2 years the child is happy just pushing a toy on wheels or carrying objects here and there. Once the child is safely on his feet, he enjoys sitting astride a wooden toy and pushing himself along with his feet. Other favourite activities are those which involve putting in and taking out, whether it is a nest of cups or the contents of the kitchen cupboard. Children play happily on their own at this age and are not old enough to co-operate with each other. They enjoy games with adults such as naming objects, rhymes to actions, looking at a picture book or throwing a ball.

Developing an identity and asserting independence

The child learns many new skills during his second year which enable him to be more independent. He can drink from a cup, he learns to feed himself with a spoon by 18 months, to help with dressing and undressing by the time he is 2 years old and he may be toilet trained during the day.

However his limitations frustrate him and his feelings are strong and urgent. He may try pushing or pulling his barrow which is stuck behind the table leg but quickly gives up and cries with frustration, at the same time refusing help because he wants to be independent.

With a new awareness of his personal identity and his own power, the 1-year-old goes through periods of asserting his own will and the word 'No' never seems to be off his lips. Confrontation with the toddler is best avoided and the situation is usually easily resolved with younger toddlers who are easily distracted.

Toilet training

By 18 months the child's nervous system is usually sufficiently developed for him to be able to interpret sensations from the bladder and to learn to control internal muscles.

Table 5.2 Developmental stages

	Freud Psychosocial stages	Piaget Cognitive stages
Infant	oral	sensorimotor 0−2 years
Toddler	anal	pre-operational 2−7 years pre-conceptual 2−4 years
Pre-schoolchild	genital	intuitive 4−7 years
Schoolchild	latent	concrete operations (early logic)
Adolescence	puberty	formal operations (logic)

When the child uses his pot he is rewarded by his mother's obvious pleasure and praise, and he is pleased and proud to give her something, the first time he has been able to do this. If his mother is completely relaxed about the procedure, ignores accidents and praises his efforts he will usually he trained quite quickly. Any anxiety in the mother is soon picked up by the child who may realise that he will gain more attention by not using the pot, and an emotionally charged situation may be the result.

Freud called this the anal stage of development in which the child learns that he can give or withhold both physically and emotionally, for example he may eat or reject food, and hand over or refuse to hand over an object, as well as using or not using his pot. Erikson, on the other hand, considered that gaining autonomy was the most important developmental task at this stage.

Most children are toilet trained by 3 years of age during the day, and by 4 years at night.

Intellectual development, birth−2 years

Piaget's theories of intellectual development consider the child's thinking in four main stages. The first stage is called the sensorimotor stage, when the baby and young toddler learn mainly through physical activity and sensory input.

The baby's initial reflex actions slowly develop into voluntary movements by trial and error. By 1 year the child will look for a toy which has been covered up because he has learnt that it still exists. In exploring his environment whether in the pram or moving around the house, the baby or toddler uses activity and all his senses to learn about the world.

2–4 YEARS

During this period the child loses his baby shape as limbs and trunk lengthen. The 2-year-old continuing to be extremely active, gains more control of his movements, for example he can kick a ball without falling over. By 3 years he can pedal his tricycle, he enjoys helping his mother with the household chores and can almost dress himself.

Increasing independence

The 2-year-old is affectionate and responsive in spite of the reputation he has for being difficult. His close attachment to his mother lessens gradually throughout this period. At first he tolerates short separations, but as he begins to appreciate that parents and others return after being absent, he accepts his parents going away more easily. The 4-year-old is very independent, and is proud of his ability to cope with everyday activities such as washing hands and dressing.

Temper tantrums

The frustration which began in the second year reaches a peak between 2 and 3 years. The child's determination to do things his way and his resistance to adult suggestions is stronger than ever but his understanding is still limited and new fears are developing, which all contribute to his anger and distress.

The child reacts physically in temper tantrums which may be provoked by unwanted adult control or minor incidents such as having to wait for his turn to choose a cake at tea-

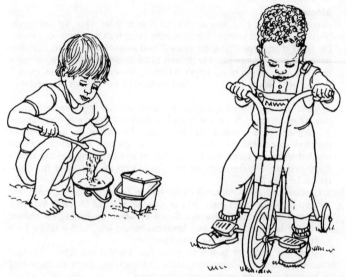

Fig. 5.8 2 years.

time, which he normally would do quite happily. The child may lie on the floor screaming and kicking. He often refuses to be comforted initially but gradually quietens enough to be lifted up and cuddled. His frustration and anger are beyond his control and his greatest fear is losing the love of his parents. He also needs the security of knowing that his parents are in control and continue to love him.

Therefore while allowing the toddler as much freedom as possible, consistent limits of behaviour set by adults provide him with the essential security which he requires.

Routine and ritual

Small children like routine and order. The 2-year-old insists on objects in the room remaining in their usual place and daily living is made into a ritual. Routine is reassuring for the child and any departure from it threatens his security and is likely to be resisted strongly.

Alexander

Alexander, aged 2½, was a cheerful little toddler who did not easily become upset and whose face constantly lit up with a mischievous smile. He liked doing everything for himself and insisted on pouring his own juice out from a large jug. He refused to be helped when using his potty and was very proud of his efforts which he showed to everyone, even if the pot was empty because he had misfired or he had not reached it in time.

Alexander had minor episodes of frustration prior to his second birthday when he could not make himself understood, but these disappeared as his speech developed. At 2½ years, he started to have temper tantrums associated with his reluctance to go out. He screamed and resisted all preparations, taking his coat off and emptying the bag which contained the requirements for the day. Once he arrived at his destination he was fine.

Certain routines in Alexander's life had to be religiously observed. He insisted on sitting in his own chair in a certain place at the table for every meal. A bedtime ritual also developed in which he had to be chased along the landing after he had been undressed and before he had his bath. The order of events was important.

Alexander had just begun to show fear for the first time. This was caused by noisy low-flying aeroplanes and dogs. In either case he rushed to his mother for protection and reassurance.

Fears and fantasies

The fears of small children arise from their vivid imaginations and their lack of understanding about cause and effect. This is Piaget's stage of pre-operational thought (2–7 years) when children do not think rationally. Some 3-year-olds really believe that they may disappear down the drain with the bath water. The child also associates his thoughts with incidents which occur at the same time, so that if his angry thoughts about his mother coincide with her going away for a few days, he assumes that he has caused her to go. The apparent power of his thoughts is terrifying and he feels guilty about what he has caused to happen. Apart from imagined fears, children have fears about real life such as the dark or walking through a wood, and they will turn to their mothers for comfort when faced with the fearful situation.

4–7 YEARS

The child seems to grow up between 3 and 4 years and no longer looks like a toddler. The 4-year-old enjoys a physical challenge such as climbing a difficult tree or a responsible job such as taking a message to a neighbour. The child is confident and more in control of his feelings though he will rush back to his parents if he is hurt or needs help. He looks up to his parents as an example, and models himself on them. His speech is grammatically correct and he knows his name and address.

By the age of 5 the child's basic personality is laid down, basic skills learnt and a pattern of relationships established. The child is ready to start school.

Broadening social horizons

Starting school involves a new routine, new activities and the prospect of meeting people without the support of parents. No wonder it is exciting but stressful. Many 5-year-olds are exhausted by the evening and need extra rest at home. The child is also relating to an adult outside the family circle for the first time and before long the child is telling his parents that 'Mrs Gray says that...' and Mrs Gray's opinion is important. However, the child continues to depend on his parents and his home to provide security, and they continue as the main influence in the child's life.

Young schoolchildren do not select a group of friends but rather work and play in loosely knit groups in which they find themselves. Children are not truly social before the age of 7 for although they play in groups, they can only co-operate by taking turns to win; this is valuable practice for true social co-operation. Quarrelling and rivalry are common between 6 and 7 years and the child's special friend one week may be banned from the house the next week. Some children who tend to be on their own, require a sensitive approach when being encouraged to join in, for children can be very cruel at this age.

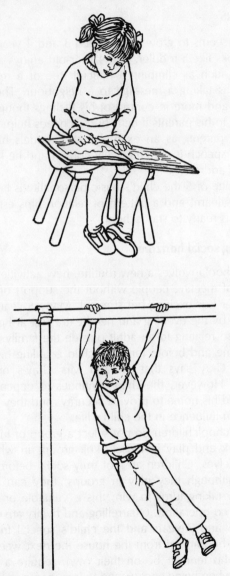

Fig. 5.9 5–6 years.

The age of individuality and self-assurance

From 4 years of age individual differences between children become increasingly apparent. Once he has gained confidence in school, the child develops a sense of power. Statements such as 'Look what I've made' or 'See how high I can climb' may sound bumptious but this is not the case for he needs encouragement to boost his self-confidence. His parents' interest and praise are essential to help him build up a sense of self-worth, which is dependent on his parents' and others' views of him. His energies may need to be channelled into constructive activities or he may turn to less desirable activities like throwing his sister's much loved doll about.

The 7-year-old is active and noisy. However when he is occupied, for example drawing a picture, he is totally absorbed, determined to draw a perfect picture which necessitates much rubbing out. For the first time he is concerned about other people's view of him and may worry about how well he will cope with what he has to do.

Intellectual development

Between 4 and 7 years the child remains egocentric, but nevertheless more aware of others and their opinion of him. Fantasies may persist until around 7 years, often as a temporary defence against reality which is sometimes too uncomfortable to face, for example when the child cannot bear to lose in a game. Wishful thinking is so strong that the wish becomes real and in any case the 6-year-old does not understand that rules are fixed, so they may be twisted to suit the circumstances. The child is gradually learning to accept himself as he is but this takes time.

The widening view of the child's world is reflected in his questions which begin with 'why', 'what for' and 'how'. This is Piaget's intuitive stage of thinking when the child may be able to group and classify objects correctly but cannot explain how he has done it, and remains unable to reason beyond his visual impressions. The following demonstration illustrates this:

Nicola
Two similar jars which contained the same amount of water were placed in front of Nicola, aged 5 years, and she agreed that the amount was the same in each. She then watched while the water from one jar was poured into a small squat jar and the water from the other jar was poured into a tall thin jar. She was then asked if the amount of water in each of these new containers was the same or different. She replied without hesitation that there was more water in the tall thin jar.

Nicola's answer was based on what she saw and the amount looked greater in the tall thin jar.

School lessons for this age group are geared to learning concepts such as 'same' and 'different' in activities which involve matching, grouping and sorting. The child learns the alphabet and progresses to reading, and learns about grouping in numbers. By 7 years the child is starting to make judgements on the basis of reasoning (not necessarily correct) rather than what he sees.

Between 4 and 7 years the child accepts other people's standards, and his developing conscience is based on his parents' attitudes. Before this age, he understands being good or being naughty but has no concept of right and wrong. Now he begins to feel bad about being naughty and by 8 years he feels shame and guilt.

7–12 YEARS

This is a healthy age when children eat well, sleep well and enjoy life. By 8 years the child's head is 90% of its adult size and children double in strength between 6 and 11 years. They are constantly on the move and dislike long periods of inactivity. Fine movements, co-ordination and stamina are improving steadily, and children enjoy using these new abilities in team sports in which social co-operation is also required. By 11 years girls are 2 years ahead of the boys developmentally.

The age of socialisation

Another name for this period is the 'primitive man' stage because children now learn to live with others and to co-operate fully with each other. The younger children play happily in a group without noticing whether members are boys or girls, but at 8 to 9 years they separate into single sex groups. The older ones begin to practise adult roles in the gangs in which they play. They enjoy real life pastimes such as fishing, reading, riding, sport or phoning their friends. They discuss matters seriously with their friends and although they can now accept that other people have different views from their own, only at around 12 years do they understand another person's point of view.

Conforming and judging

Children's increasing sensitivity to the opinion of other children is related to their desire to be accepted by their own age group. They want to conform to the standards of the group or gang, and this includes being similarly dressed whether in school uniform or leisure wear, behaving and talking in the same way as well as knowing the 'in' jokes, and the secret language. As parents know only too well, their opinions on what the child should wear are not accepted as they previously were, although parents continue to influence the child. Children no longer consider adults infallible and start to make judgements, for example on their teacher. The handicapped child of this age may have a difficult time if he is unable to join in physical activities or to conform to some of the rules of the gang.

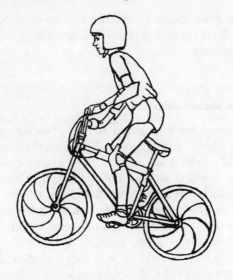

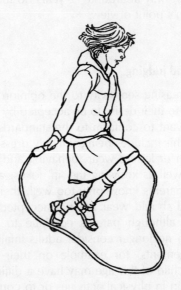

Fig. 5.10 7–12 years.

The beginning of logical thinking

Piaget calls this the stage of concrete operations. The child begins to think logically and to use logic in solving problems but only if he can see them in front of him. Problems must be factual and concrete, hence the name of this stage. The child understands cause and effect and looks for reasons. He can group and classify accurately and enjoys sorting objects into a logical order. Children practise this in a popular pastime for this age group, collecting anything from matchboxes to shells.

During the middle school years the child enjoys learning and is interested in schoolwork. He uses words more effectively and his knowledge increases rapidly. He asks more searching questions and understands more complicated explanations. The older child understands time and space in its wider sense and is able to consider events outside his own experience, so geography and history interest him. By 12 years the child is progressing towards patterns of adult thinking.

ADOLESCENCE

Puberty is the period when sexual organs and secondary sex characteristics develop. It begins with a growth spurt with maximum growth of girls around 12 years and of boys around 14 years. Adolescence is the stage of development in which the child becomes a young adult. It begins at puberty and most people consider it to end at around 18 years. However some experts consider that this stage is not complete by 18 years and a few suggest that 25 years would be more accurate.

During adolescence the individual is developing an identity of his own. In doing this he is learning to be independent and to accept himself as he is. He thinks about his role in society, the type of work he would like to do and the values on which he bases his attitudes, behaviour and moral judgements.

A sense of identity

The young adolescent has a heightened awareness of himself. He is often self-conscious about his changing body shape, sensitive to other people's opinion of him and self-critical. Moving towards adulthood is challenging but brings new responsibilities for which he may not feel prepared, so that he has swings of mood between elation and uncertainty.

Adolescents need to develop an identity so that they can accept themselves, and to appreciate that they are lovable and worthy. This is largely dependent on attitudes of friends and parents who can boost morale and give the young person confidence.

Independence

At times the adolescent behaves like a child, dependent and helpless, whereas at others he is responsible and co-operative. He has strong drives to be independent yet sometimes needs as much support as a child.

In this transitional stage, it is also difficult for his parents to relinquish control yet maintain their support. The adolescent's mood swings make the parents unsure how best to relate to him, for he may be rude, resentful and unco-operative. He is certainly likely to criticise them, challenge their authority, to argue about times for returning home and to be secretive about his activities. His parents worry about his safety, his involvement with the opposite sex and the influence of the peer group who may encourage him to participate in activities such as drug taking.

A social role

By the mid-teens the adolescent is more influenced by the opinions and rules of the gang than by his parents' requests. His or her hairstyle, dress and other distinguishing features may stretch parents' tolerance to the limit but they are evidence of belonging, which is important. The group provides mutual support, friendship and a forum for discussing common difficulties in a sympathetic environment free from criticism and conflict. It also helps the adolescent to make the break from the family and to become more independent.

Intellectual maturity

The 12-year-old is starting to develop adult patterns of thinking and by 15 years is capable of formal logic and solving abstract problems. He is able to reason deductively, and evaluate and criticise his own thinking. In school work hypotheses are formulated, tested and evaluated.

Sex role identity

The adolescent moves through various types of relationships to become a young adult who is capable of a range of feelings from friendly indifference to deep involvement with a member of the opposite sex.

The single sex groups of the 10- to 12-year-olds continue into early adolescence and at the same time 'crushes' on older people, pop stars or athletes are common. Gradually this changes to an interest in those of the opposite sex, a stage which girls reach first, for their development remains 2 years ahead at this age.

Early relationships between boys and girls are usually in groups rather than pairs. In the mid- or late teens the adolescent may then pass through a series of short-lived one-to-one relationships with the opposite sex before a friendship develops into a mature long-term relationship.

Into work

A worthwhile occupation means more than working for economic ends. It should provide self-fulfilment and self-respect, in other words job satisfaction.

The teenager is under considerable pressure with examinations to take, his future to think about, a job to organise or further education to arrange. Doubts and uncertainties within himself and problems in society such as a high rate of unemployment, do not make it any easier for him. He needs to make his own decisions about his future but at the same time requires support and guidance from parents and teachers.

A philosophy of life

A reference framework for religious, political and philosophical views is developed in the late teens or early 20s. The young adult questions his own ideas on these matters, which he previously accepted from his parents, and often challenges the established order.

The young person may pass through a phase of total dedication to a political or social cause and be idealistic and intolerant of the double standards which he sees in society or in his family. Parents have little control over their children at this stage, although many of them continue to turn to their parents when they want something! This is usually a sympathetic ear, tolerant understanding or financial help.

REFERENCES AND FURTHER READING

Altschul A T 1975 Psychology for nurses. Baillière Tindall, London, chs 2–5
Erikson E 1977 Childhood and society. Triad/Paladin, London
Hadfield J A 1975 Childhood and adolescence. Penguin, Harmondsworth
Holt K S 1977 Developmental paediatrics. Butterworth, London
Illingworth R S 1983 The normal child, 8th edn. Churchill Livingstone, Edinburgh
Illingworth R S 1977 Basic developmental screening 0–2 years. Blackwell, Oxford
Sheridan M D 1975 Children's developmental progress from birth to five years. NFER, Windsor, Berks
Whaley L F, Wong D L 1981 Nursing care of infants and children. C. V. Mosby, St Louis

Primary health care
    team
    Health visitor
School health service
    and role of school
    nurse
The handicapped child
    at home
    The handicapped
        infant

District handicap
    team
Paediatric assessment
    unit
Parents of
    handicapped or
    chronically ill
    children
Community mental
    handicap nurse

6

Child health in the community

PRIMARY HEALTH CARE TEAM

The primary health care team is the family's initial point of contact with the health service. The team consists of the general practitioner, the health visitor, the district nurse and her team, and sometimes a midwife and social worker. In addition to the doctor's daily surgery, clinics and occasionally meetings are organised for specific groups of clients. Antenatal care, family planning, 'well-woman' checks, and child health clinics may all be organised in this way.

Child health clinics are run by the health visitor who monitors the child's development and progress, and the general practitioner who sees the child at intervals or if there is a problem. Immunisations are carried out and mothers are given advice and support.

Some child health clinics, which are held in church halls or similar places, are organised by the local health authority for families in a geographic area. These work on similar lines, with a health visitor, and a doctor who is appointed by the local authority. Mothers can buy infant foods there and in a few clinics additional facilities are provided such as a toy library or treatment for minor disorders.

Table 6.1 Immunisation programme from birth to 4 years

Age	Immunisation	
Neonate	BCG	infants of Asian mothers or with family history of tuberculosis
3 months	Diphtheria Pertussis DPT Tetanus	1st dose
5 months	DPT Poliomyelitis	2nd dose
10 months	DPT Poliomyelitis	3rd dose
1 year	Measles	

HEALTH VISITOR (HV)

The HV, by promoting health and health policies, empowers people to take responsibility for health as individuals, families and communities, thereby helping to prevent and minimise the effects of disease, dysfunction and disability.

Health Visitor Association 1985

This definition of the health visitor's role is a good one in that it shows that health visitors are primarily proactive. They search out and stimulate an awareness of health needs by identifying health-damaging behaviour such as having an inadequate diet, and encouraging individuals to change this. They help to initiate change by, for example, identifying a group with particular needs such as isolated women on a large housing estate, and then working with them to set up a support network. The HV is essentially a family visitor who is a first line of defence in that she goes into people's homes when there is not necessarily any problem.

A typical day in the life of a HV is described here in order to illustrate the diversity of the work.

Development assessment

The day starts with a visit to Jimmy, a 2-year-old who is due for his development check. This is the backbone of health visiting—routine assessments of babies and children under 5 years, looking at their physical, social and emotional development at specific times in their lives, in order to prevent or to detect potential problems early.

The HV has known Jimmy and his family since he was a baby, having seen him at regular intervals throughout that time. She knows that he can be quite a handful. She not only wants to see how Jimmy is, but also to see how his mother is coping with the 'terrible twos'.

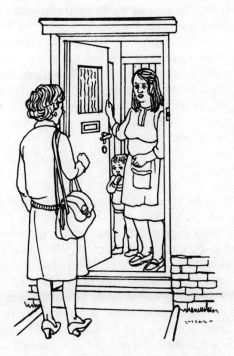

Fig. 6.1 The health visitor supports and advises parents in their own homes.

The knock on the door is almost drowned by Jimmy's shouts and a loud crash. Mrs Ball looks harrassed as she answers the door. Jimmy has just climbed on to the sideboard and broken a favourite ornament. The health visitor and Mrs Ball discuss Jimmy's difficult behaviour and conclude that he is probably bored. While talking about various solutions, Mrs Ball decides that taking him to a mother and toddler group at the local clinic might help. She also wants to discuss toilet training, as Jimmy is starting to show some awareness of what is happening in that direction. The health visitor also feels it may be an appropriate time to talk about home safety, as Jimmy's climbing skills could clearly get him into trouble. She and Mrs Ball discuss fire guards, safety gates and where to store medicines and household chemicals.

Throughout the visit, the health visitor has been noting Jimmy's use of language, his physical skills in moving around as well as in building bricks and scribbling. She has also talked with his mother about diet and sleeping. She arranges to return in 3 months time to see if Jimmy's behaviour has become any easier to handle. She makes sure that Mrs Ball has the health centre telephone number to ring should she want the health visitor to call.

New baby

The health visitor next calls on Mr and Mrs Wright and their first baby who is 11 days old. She first met the family when Mrs Wright was pregnant and has since seen her regularly at home and at the GP's antenatal clinic. The midwife, who has been visiting Mrs Wright daily since her discharge from hospital, may continue to visit up to 28 days, and may contact the health visitor in order to exchange any relevant information. The health visitor will decide how often the Wrights need her to visit, probably weekly initially then less frequently as the baby gets older. Mr Wright had a week off work to help his wife and has now gone back to his job.

Mrs Wright feels rather alone and unsure although she tries to put on a bright and cheery appearance when the health visitor calls. The health visitor examines the baby and talks to Mrs Wright about her main worries which are the baby's feeds and how much the baby should be sleeping. They also discuss the baby's immunisations, particularly in the light of the current whooping cough epidemic. Mrs Wright has heard stories about brain damage and needs information and reassurance.

Gradually the health visitor leads the conversation round to Mrs Wright herself, emphasising the importance of looking after her health and wellbeing. It eventually emerges that Mrs Wright has been feeling very weepy, particularly since her husband's return to work. The health visitor discusses the problem with her and arranges to call back in 2 days time.

Visiting the elderly

The health visitor has received a message from the liaison health visitor for the geriatric wards at the local hospital about Mr Evans who is 82 years old. She calls to assess his situation and to see that he is managing on his own. The elderly are an important client group for health visitors.

Social problem

The school nurse who works in the same office as the health visitor has told her about a 9-year-old boy, Alan Dawes, who is always smelly and unkempt at school. She thinks he might be wetting the bed and wonders if there are problems at home. The health visitor knows the family well and remembers Alan as a little boy so she arranges to visit his home to ascertain if they have problems. She recalls that his father was a labourer and as unemployment in the area over the last few years has risen, the health visitor wonders if Alan's father has been laid off and whether this may have anything to do with Alan's appearance at school.

Both Mr and Mrs Dawes are at home when the health visitor calls and both look depressed. In conversation the health visitor discovers that Mr Dawes was made redundant 3 months ago and they are finding it very difficult to manage financially. The conversation turns to welfare benefits and the health visitor is able to advise on what the family is able to claim. Their money worries have been affecting their relationship and Alan has been picking up the friction between them, which is probably why he has been wetting the bed. The health visitor refers Alan to the enuresis clinic at the health centre and discusses making a star chart for Alan as a system of rewards for a dry bed. Both Mr and Mrs Dawes seem relieved that there is something they can do. She invites Mrs Dawes to a women's group which is being held regularly at the local community centre.

Health education

The health visitor returns to the health centre in order to write up the visits she has carried out that day and to make the necessary telephone calls and referrals. She also needs to look over the material for the Open University course on the pre-school child which she runs one evening a week. This is for a group of women who have been experiencing various problems with their toddlers. The course has been running for 4 weeks and although at first the women had been loath to say much their confidence has been increasing over the weeks, and now the health visitor has difficulty getting a word in. The women have said that the course material and the chance to talk to other mothers have given them a greater insight into their own children's behaviour.

Child abuse

In the middle of this paper work, the health visitor receives a telephone call from the local nursery. A 3-year-old girl has been found to have a strange bruise on the side of her face and the nursery teacher asks the health visitor to come and look at it. She goes immediately to the nursery and examines the child. The mark looks as though it has been the result of an intentional injury so the health visitor follows a set procedure for action when child abuse is suspected. She tells the nursery teacher that as it is nearly time for the child's mother to collect her, she will wait, talk to the mother and then arrange for the child to be seen by the doctor at the health centre. In the meantime she telephones the nursing officer to report the incident and also contacts the social worker who has been dealing with the family.

When the mother is asked about the bruise, she first of all says that the child fell against the table and then that her young son hit her. Neither the doctor nor the social worker are happy with the varying accounts so a decision is made to take the mother and child to the hospital where she can be examined by a paediatrician. While these decisions are being made, the health visitor is quietly talking with the mother who breaks down and admits that she hit the little girl because she had spilled her dinner. There is clearly a great deal of stress in the family, and the health visitor reassures the mother that she will receive the help and support she needs. When the mother and child have gone to the hospital the HV returns to the health centre to write a report about the incident, which is also recorded in the child's documents.

The handicapped child

Finally before the HV leaves the health centre, the mother of a 4-year-old child with hemiplegia telephones to talk about the child's behaviour and to seek reassurance that she is 'doing the right thing' in being firm with her.

The developmental checks which the HV carries out in the child's home and in the clinic enable her to detect early signs of handicap so that the child can be referred to a paediatrician for further assessment without delay. When a child's handicap is identified, the HV can help by being available and supporting the family, working with them at their pace and putting them in touch with the right people at the right time. She may help with aids, adaptations to the house and claiming welfare benefits. She may also put the family in touch with other parents in a support group.

The end of the day

The health visitor's day has been a busy but satisfying one. Not all days are so satisfying, when families are out and several calls may be required before she finds them in. While most clients accept the health visitor's advice gratefully, some refuse to do so. The HV continues to support these families as best she can.

SCHOOL HEALTH SERVICE AND ROLE OF SCHOOL NURSE

The function of the school health service is to safeguard the health of the schoolchild and to ensure that he is as fit as possible in order to obtain the maximum benefit from his education. The school team includes the doctor, nurse, dentist, technician and other professional staff who visit the school occasionally. The child's first and main contact with the service is through the school nurse and school medical officer. The child with a problem which necessitates further investigation or treatment is referred to his family doctor, a hospital or a specialist clinic.

Routine examinations

The school nurse performs various screening tests throughout the child's school years, and assists the school doctor with medical examinations and immunisation clinics.

The following schedule is a typical programme:

Age	Examination
4½–5 years	Medical examination including squint test
	Immunisation against diphtheria, tetanus and polio
	Hearing and vision tests
8–10 years	Medical examination if there is a potential problem or if parents request it
	Immunisation if necessary
	Hearing screening test by audiometrician
	Vision screening test by technician
10 years	Immunisation against rubella (girls only)
	Screening for scoliosis—back inspection annually until leaving school (girls only)
11 years	Tuberculosis testing and BCG immunisation if necessary
12 years	Vision screening test, including colour vision
13 years	Vision screening test
14–15 years	Medical review by the doctor
	Immunisation booster against tetanus and polio
	Vision screening test
	Blood pressure recorded
	Urinalysis.

In addition to these examinations, the school nurse sees all the children individually each year.

The parents' permission is obtained for all examinations or immunisations and before the child is referred for any further treatment. Parents are encouraged to attend their child's medical examinations, they are notified about any disorder and asked to ensure that any necessary treatment is undertaken.

The school doctor and nurse work closely with teaching colleagues and social workers when necessary, helping children with social, emotional, learning and medical problems. The child with learning problems may be referred to the educational psychologist.

Craig

Craig was 11 years old and grossly overweight. He weighed in at 84 kilograms, more than twice the average for his age. His parents owned a fish and chip shop and did nothing to encourage him to lose weight. He experienced many problems at school from slowness in moving about and difficulty in participating in sport to comments and ridicule from his classmates.

Craig's problem was discussed with his parents over a period of 9 months before they would agree to his referral to a paediatrician. He was admitted to the ward so that his food intake could be controlled. The family were fully involved and the importance of their role was discussed with them. Craig started to lose weight immediately on his restricted diet and after 2 weeks of satisfactory progress he was discharged home, confident that he could keep to his diet. Shortly after this, the family moved away and no follow-up was possible.

Obesity is notoriously difficult to treat successfully, more so when parents are overweight themselves and not convinced that it matters. With this background and without regular follow-up and the support which it provides, Craig would probably relapse to his former weight.

Screening tests

Screening procedures lead to early diagnosis and treatment of disorders of growth or of any aspect of development. Scoliosis affects mainly girls and therefore screening is limited to females. The curvature of the spine which it causes, increases rapidly during adolescence and may lead to cardiac and respiratory complications. Major surgery is required for advanced cases.

Following the schedule previously described, screening for defects in vision and hearing is carried out at regular intervals.

Lyndsay

Lyndsay, aged 5 years, was found to have little vision in one eye when she had her routine vision test on school entry. Her parents had not noticed her having any difficulty in seeing and Lyndsay had never complained because, as far as she knew, her view of the world was normal. After a visit to the optician and the provision of spectacles, a whole new world opened up for her.

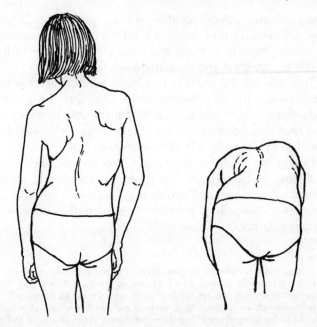

Fig. 6.2 Screening for scoliosis. A spinal curvature is present and does not disappear when the child bends forward.

Health care interviews

The school nurse sees each child individually at least once a year and each term if the child has any kind of problem. These interviews have developed from the former hygiene inspections which most people remember for the great emphasis which was placed on the checking of children's hair for head lice and nits. The school nurse tended to be associated with this aspect, hence her nickname 'Nitty Nora' or 'the nit nurse'.

In the health care interview the nurse takes into consideration every aspect of the child's life, using any opportunity which arises for health education. The child's height and weight are measured annually and recorded on a centile chart, which helps to identify children who are failing to thrive. Children whose names are on the child abuse register or where there is a strong suspicion of child abuse in the family are weighed and measured each term.

To overcome the problem of infested heads which has not gone away, the nurse spends more time with the parents individually and in groups, teaching them how to recognise and deal with the problem. It is not unknown for one-third of the class in a primary school to have head lice.

During the interview the child is free to talk about any problems he has. These may relate to schoolwork, family difficulties or emotional problems. The nurse may act as counsellor especially to the older ones who often bring their problems to her.

Wayne

During a health interview Wayne, aged 12 years, appeared to the nurse to be abnormally anxious about moving to the local high school in 9 months time. This was obviously preying on his mind for he voiced his fears without any prompting. It seemed early in the school year for a child to be so concerned. He also complained about attacks of feeling hot in the classroom and said that he was having a lot of headaches. He had been absent from school for 1 or 2 days but his teachers were unaware of any problem.

The school nurse helped Wayne by listening to him and encouraging him to talk, so that he was able to identify two areas of school life which worried him. These were discussed with the doctor and his teacher who were able to help him, once they understood his difficulties.

Wayne's anxiety and his physical symptoms might have been early signs of school refusal or phobia. He was able to overcome his problem with the help he received, but if his condition had deteriorated further, he would have been referred to a child psychiatrist for specialist help.

Dental inspection

Dental inspections and treatment are carried out by the community dental service at regular intervals, usually annually. Parents may use this service or alternatively may take their children to their own family dentist. Some schools are visited by fully equipped dental trailers enabling the treatment to be given at the school.

Speech therapists

Most areas have peripatetic speech therapists who help children with speech problems reported by teaching or medical staff. They hold speech therapy sessions in schools and local clinics.

Handicapped children

The school health service is closely involved with children with special educational needs which includes those with a handicap. Children are assessed when they enter school, and at other times to check their progress or when they are due to move to another school. The school doctor supervises these children closely, paying attention to their disability as well as their progress in school. At times he may need to contact colleagues to discuss problems or to organise help from other agencies.

Some children with special needs require frequent attention from the school nurse, such as regular medication or treatment. Children may also need help at unpredictable times, for example with a difficult caliper or a hearing aid which is not working. Where there is a unit for handicapped children and in special schools, additional staff and facilities are required.

The school nurse can help the handicapped child and his teacher by explaining to her about the handicap and the problems which it creates for the child. The teacher should be given essential knowledge about any aspects which might require action from her, such as the child having an epileptic fit, and the parents may wish to be involved with this. The teacher probably needs support, as well as encouragement not to overprotect the child. The rest of the class should have some understanding of the child's difficulties and be taught to accept the child on equal terms without pity or teasing.

Health education

Health education is inherent in many of the duties of the school nurse. Advising the mother of a 4-year-old about treating her child's infested hair, discussing skin care with a spotty adolescent, or chatting with a handicapped 10-year-old about school dinners may all provide opportunities for health education at a time when the recipient is interested and receptive to advice.

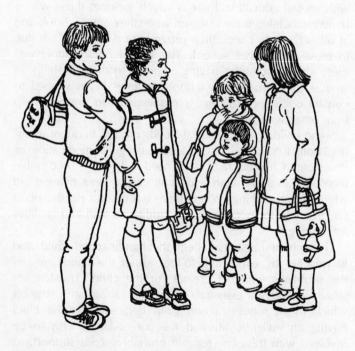

Fig. 6.3 School provides many opportunities for health education.

The school doctor and nurse see the parents when they attend their children's routine examinations. The nurse may visit the child's home to discuss a problem which has been identified at school or to check that the child's treatment, for example for enuresis, is being carried out correctly. These contacts enable health topics to be mentioned quite naturally in the course of conversation and much valuable advice may be given at these times.

Health education is an established part of the school curriculum. The school nurse may take occasional sessions but the teachers are responsible for most of the teaching and for integrating the material in many different subjects. Literature is now available for teachers both on the organisation of a health education programme and on the content. A structured and co-ordinated approach is used which the teachers can adapt to suit their own situation.

THE HANDICAPPED CHILD AT HOME

Most handicapped children are cared for in the community by their parents. A handicap may be physical or mental or the child may be multiply handicapped. It is important to think of the child with a handicap as a normal individual who happens to have a handicap rather than as a handicapped child, which places the emphasis on the handicap first and the child second. The mentally handicapped child's intelligence may be at any level from just below average to the lowest level of severe subnormality, incapable of living an independent life. A different approach is required for each child.

THE HANDICAPPED INFANT

Early identification of a handicap gives the child the best chance of achieving his potential. For example, parents of a baby who is blind from birth require instruction early in the first year on how to stimulate their baby by non-visual methods, providing a selection of toys which encourage normal development and bring the child out of himself. Peripatetic teachers of the blind visit the home and give specialist advise and support. Likewise the earlier the mentally handicapped child is identified, the sooner training programmes can be established to minimise developmental delay.

DISTRICT HANDICAP TEAM

Previously the handicapped child's care involved supervision and treatment by numerous professional staff, which resulted in frequent visits to hospital, conflicting advice and confused parents. Co-ordination of care of handicapped children has improved where district handicap teams have been set up to provide a link between the families, staff and relevant services. A paediatrician, nurse or health visitor, a social worker and an educational psychologist form the basis of this multi-disciplinary team although many other specialists are involved. The district handicap team gives information, support and advice to parents, teachers and other professional staff who are involved in the care of handicapped children. It also advises on specific children with special problems and works to improve facilities and training of staff.

PAEDIATRIC ASSESSMENT UNIT

Children under the age of 5 years are often assessed in paediatric assessment units. The child attends with his mother for several days so that he can be fully assessed in every aspect of development, and in different situations such as at play and mealtimes. Each member of the unit's multi-disciplinary team examines the child, and his mother also makes a valuable contribution to the assessment. At the end of the week the team meet to discuss their individual findings and produce a report. The child's problems and needs are identified and decisions made about treatment and continuing care. Plans are fully discussed with the child's parents and they are given a copy of the report.

Key worker

A named member of the team is designated as the key worker. This person ensures that all aspects of the child's care are integrated. She keeps in touch with the family and is available at any time should they have a problem or want to talk to someone. The pre-school child with poor concentration or a speech defect may attend the paediatric assessment unit for individual or group therapy. Advice is also given on feeding or other difficulties, and equipment can be borrowed for home use. Parent groups are popular and provide them with opportunities to discuss their problems, exchange ideas and to gain support from each other.

Special educational needs

The Warnock Report (1978) recommended that educational provision for children with special problems such as physical or mental handicap, learning difficulty or psychiatric disorder, should be based on their educational needs rather than on the type of handicap. The report also suggested that these children should be educated in ordinary schools as far as possible. Many of these recommendations have been incorporated into the 1981 Education Act (England and Wales). One of the main purposes of assessing handicapped schoolchildren is to ensure that they receive the most appropriate schooling for them. An annual assessment is recommended so that the child can be moved from one school to another as his needs change.

Which school?

There are several methods of integrating children with special educational needs into ordinary schools. The bright physically handicapped child may manage in an ordinary school without difficulty if the building is adapted. Some handicapped children may join an ordinary class for part of the day, and slow learners may be withdrawn temporarily from an ordinary class to a remedial group. Special facilities, such as treatment rooms where incontinent children can change, are required for many handicapped children. A problem which often worries school staff is the child who may need emergency treatment, for example the diabetic who may become hypoglycaemic.

Severely handicapped children do well at special schools which have extra facilities and specially trained teachers. A disadvantage is the isolation of the handicapped children from their normal peers, which deprives them of opportunities of learning to mix and make friends in a situation which they will have to face when they leave school.

PARENTS OF HANDICAPPED OR CHRONICALLY ILL CHILDREN

The care and treatment of a handicapped child is largely dependent on the parents, as it is for a child with a long-term or chronic illness. The parents are responsible for the child's daily care and maintaining any treatment or training programme. They also understand the child better than anyone else.

Feelings and problems

Adjusting to having a handicapped or chronically sick child is difficult, because of the many reactions and strong feelings which may surface at different times. A stressful time for parents is when they are first told about the child's problem, whether this is at birth or later. The parents are likely to have feelings of denial, anger, and guilt, grieving for the normal child they have lost. Telling the family and friends can pose problems and maintaining normal family life may not be easy but is important for the child and the other children.

Daily care may be time consuming and exhausting, and curtailment of social life leading to social isolation may cause stress and affect relationships within the family. Extra expense is often incurred, holidays or even arranging a break from caring for the child may be difficult. Parents may feel irritable, unable to cope, tired, frustrated and anxious about the child's future.

Help for parents

Parents are helped by being involved with the child's assessment and treatment, by regular contact maintained with professional staff and the availability of help in an emergency. They should know all about the child's condition, treatment, future plans and his prognosis. Counselling may help them to work through their feelings, with additional support at stressful times such as when the child changes school, has an operation, is re-admitted to hospital or the parents are told that his condition has deteriorated. Practical help and support are provided by community or hospital staff. The handicapped child may be admitted to hospital to give the mother a break and the social worker can help with holiday arrangements. She can also help the parents to apply for the benefits to which they are entitled.

COMMUNITY MENTAL HANDICAP NURSE (CMHN)

The CMHN is a member of the community mental handicap team which enables families to care for a mentally handicapped child or adult at home. This description of how the CMHN helped Paul and his parents demonstrates the value of continuity of care by one keyworker.

Paul

Paul was 7 years old when he was referred to the community mental handicap team. He was born physically and mentally handicapped and had never walked. However he managed to move around on his knees and his mother took him out in a pushchair for he had insufficient strength to control a wheelchair. He was prone to severe chest infections and he also suffered from epilepsy, which was well controlled except when he had an infection. He could not speak but made a few noises and his parents had always given him liquidised food because they thought he might choke on hard or lumpy foods.

The nurse who looked after Paul visited every 3 or 4 weeks and spent the first 18 months building up a relationship with the family and supporting them through a difficult time. Paul had glandular fever for one school term, and just as he was recovering his father developed reactive depression. This lasted for 6 months and no changes were possible during this time.

After 18 months of regular visiting and discussion about Paul learning to eat solid foods, his parents finally agreed to a trial.

A training programme

The nurse first asked the parents to help her to complete an assessment of Paul's strengths and weaknesses using the Portage checklist, which they were happy to do. Devised in the USA, the Portage scheme requires the participation of parents to assess the abilities of mentally handicapped children up to 6 years of age, according to such categories as socialisation, language, self-help and cognitive aspects.

Assessing Paul's feeding with his parents, the nurse recorded his position for feeding (sitting in own chair), method (spoon fed), food (liquids), social interaction (nil). She then wrote an activity chart with the procedure of feeding divided into small steps which would eventually wean Paul onto a varied diet of solid food, thus achieving the goal.

On the first occasion he ate a biscuit which he enjoyed and took without any problem. His parents were much more enthusiastic after this first major hurdle had been overcome. He then progressed to grated apple and grated carrot, each new taste being introduced several days after the previous one. Because his parents feared that he might choke, the nurse remained with the family when they tried a new food, but there were no problems. Paul could now feed himself part of his diet using his fingers which was an important step towards greater independence.

Paul continued to increase his intake of solid food and his progress was obvious on his chart which thrilled his parents. Paul was also learning to pull himself up, so he might eventually be able to walk.

The role of the community mental handicap nurse

The nurse acts as co-ordinator between the family and other professionals, she assesses the child's needs and initiates training programmes for the parents to implement. Parents can telephone the nurse if they are worried, and she may accompany the child and his mother on their visits to hospital clinics. The nurse may obtain toys for them but often advises on better use of toys and items already available in the home. She can also obtain enuresis alarms, feeding and incontinence aids. The CMHN reports back to the team at a weekly meeting when members discuss clients' progress and exchange ideas on dealing with problems which have arisen.

The community mental handicap nurse has undertaken a basic 3 year course to become a Registered Nurse for Mental Handicap. There is an 18 month post-registration course in this speciality for RGN nurses and a 1 year course for RMN nurses. A further course for those intending to work in the community is the ENB Course 805 on community nursing in mental handicap.

REFERENCES AND FURTHER READING

Health visiting and school nursing
Keywood O 1982 Personal and community health. Blackwell, Oxford, chs 9, 10, 11
Turton P, Orr J 1985 Learning to care in the community. Hodder and Stoughton, London

The handicapped child
Finnie N R 1974 Handling the young cerebral palsied child at home. Heinemann, London
General Nursing Council 1982 Aspects of sick children's nursing: a learning package. GNC for England and Wales (now English National Board), London, Study Units 40–44
Newsom J, Newsom E 1979 Toys and playthings. Allen and Unwin, London
Polney L, Hull D 1985 Community paediatrics. Churchill Livingstone, Edinburgh
Warnock H M (Chairman) 1978 Special education needs. The report of the Committee of Enquiry into the Educational Needs of Handicapped Children and Young People. HMSO, London

PART | THREE

Practical aspects of children's care

Maintaining a safe
   environment
   Safety in the ward
   Infection
   Administration of
     medicines and
     injections
   Cardiac arrest
Body temperature
   Practical procedures

Care of the pyrexial
   child
   Febrile convulsions
Breathing
   Assessment and
     identification of
     problems
   Practical procedures
   Care of the baby with
     bronchiolitis
   Croup

7

A safe environment, body temperature, breathing

MAINTAINING A SAFE ENVIRONMENT

Dependence on others is one of the characteristics of children which makes them different from adults. From the infant's total dependence the child gradually moves towards independence but even older sensible children require some supervision. Taking over the care of other people's children is not easy and paediatric staff are very aware of their responsibility for the children's safety. This burden is reduced in hospital wards when parents are resident or present for most of the day.

The law allows people to give consent for their own treatment when they reach 16 years of age, but the adolescent is not necessarily ready to make such decisions and continues to need support. Mentally handicapped children require constant supervision regardless of their age.

SAFETY IN THE WARD

Safety includes psychological safety, that is providing an

emotionally secure environment for the child. This aspect is discussed in Chapter 2. Physical safety in hospital involves high standards of care, for instance using a correct aseptic technique for applying a dressing, conscientious hand-washing and safety precautions in basic care, for instance never moving away from a baby in a cot with the side down.

For the child to be allowed as much freedom as possible in the ward, it must be a safe place for children. A high staff/patient ratio is required to supervise them and there should always be an adult in the ward; parents often help the staff in this. An observant nurse may be able to anticipate which children are liable to get into mischief. It is usually the active, the hyperactive, the inquisitive toddler or the child who is bored. The child can ruin the best planned care of the nurse quite innocently.

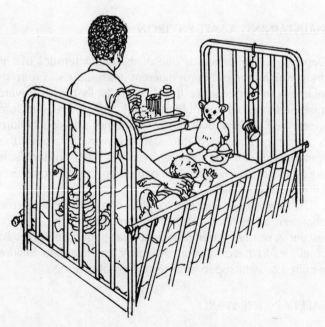

Fig. 7.1 Keep a hand on the baby when turning away from the cot.

Lucy

Lucy arrived in the anaesthetic room for her tonsillectomy drowsy but comfortable. She was found to have the remains of a chocolate biscuit in her mouth. A short while before, in the ward, the cleaner had moved the cots and beds in order to clean the floor and Lucy's cot had ended up near another child's locker on which were some biscuits. Lucy who was very hungry had made the most of this opportunity. The incident was over in a few minutes and no-one had noticed.

Some of the hazards in the children's ward

Hazard	Safety measure
Building	
Stairs	Gate at top or bottom of stairs, or both.
	Narrow gaps between bannisters to prevent toddlers passing through.
	Bannister high enough to prevent child climbing on or over.
Windows	Sealed or opening at top only, or opening at the bottom blocked at safe height.
	No furniture for climbing on near windows.
	Strengthened glass in areas where child might fall.
Treatment room, kitchen & other rooms	Doors kept closed.
	Additional high handles on doors.
	Children excluded except with adult.
	Certain cupboards locked.
Doors	Care opening doors.
	Observation panel in swing doors.
Heat/Fire	
Hot water	Hot water in tap controlled at safe level.
	Baby's feeds warmed in hot *not* boiling water.
	Hot water bottles not used. If unavoidable, fill with hot (not boiling) water and place blanket between child and bottle.
Bath water	Run cold water first, test temperature using own elbow and not child's toe.
Radiators	Correctly guarded.

Hazard	Safety measure
	Cots and beds at safe distance from radiator.
Oxygen	Sparking or metal toys banned near oxygen therapy.
	Warning notices about risk displayed clearly. Parents and visitors told.
Children Cot/bed	Child only in cot or bed when essential.
	Cotsides always fully raised.
	Never move away from child in cot with the cotside down.
	Look out for pillows or toys making steps for child to climb up and over cotside.
	Make sure the child has plenty to do.
Pillows/plastic bags	No pillows for babies under 1 year.
	If baby to be propped up, use pillows under mattress.
	No plastic bags in the ward.
	Take care with plastic pillowcovers.
Cords, strings & ties	Beware of any cord, dress tie or string on toy which could get entangled round child's neck. Remove doubtful ones.
Bathing	Do not leave toddler in the bath alone—he may slip.
Sharp objects	Remove sharp-edged badges from uniform and equipment from uniform pockets. Watch out for sharp edges of toys.
	Close napkin pin when removed while changing baby.
	Do not allow children to walk around with stick, pen or toothbrush in mouth.
Small objects for swallowing or inhaling	Remove likely objects from young children (buttons, beads, peanuts, marbles, coins).

Other hazards in the ward are those which are related to the care and treatment of patients.

Electrical sockets and electrical equipment such as fans, nebulisers and suction machines are all potential dangers. Children may be tempted to investigate them and may also damage them when playing boisterous games. Restricting the child to his bed or cot unnecessarily increases the risk of him falling out. Children are safer on the floor.

If an accident does occur the incident must be reported to the nurse in charge at once. The doctor will examine the child and an X-ray may be ordered. The parents will be informed and an incident form must be completed on the same day. This should include names of witnesses, any injuries and details about the incident, written by the person who was most involved with the accident.

INFECTION

Infection is another hazard in the children's ward. There is usually some infection, for example a respiratory infection, a streptococcal throat infection, whooping cough or an infected wound. Allocation of nurses to care for individual patients helps to reduce cross-infection.

Infants

Infants under 6 months and in some areas those under 1 year, are nursed in cubicles or in a bay separated from other children. In this way they are protected to a certain degree from infections in the ward, but the isolation in a cubicle is not good for their emotional and social development. To overcome this, parents are encouraged to stay or visit frequently and the nurse caring for the baby should make time to cuddle, talk and play with him.

Wearing plastic aprons is the most effective method of protecting the child from organisms on the nurse's dress. The apron is hung in the cubicle, and the outside (which touches the baby) should be clearly marked. Cotton gowns may be used similarly but are not bacteria-proof when damp. They may also be worn over a plastic apron. Equipment used regularly is kept in the cubicle all the time and hands should always be washed before touching the child and before leaving the cubicle. Handwashing is the single most important factor in preventing the spread of infection.

Barrier nursing

Protective nursing (or reverse isolation) has been described above in the infant's care. Barrier nursing (or source protection) is used to protect patients and staff from infectious patients. Precautions differ according to the mode of spread of the infection.

Airborne and enteric infections are probably most common. In both cases, the child with the infection should be nursed in a cubicle with the door shut. One nurse should look after the child during each shift. A plastic apron should be worn during contact with the child and hands should be washed afterwards. When in contact with secretions in an airborne infection and the excreta in an enteric infection, a plastic apron and gloves should be worn, and again hands washed afterwards.

Hands. Hands should be thoroughly washed under running water, using elbow taps correctly. The towel should be a paper one and placed in an appropriate bin after use. Handwashing is carried out on entering the cubicle, again if necessary before a clean procedure such as feeding an infant, and finally before leaving.

Equipment and clothing. Disposable equipment and clothes which can be laundered should be used. A pedal bin for waste and another bin for soiled linen and clothes are necessary and the hospital method for dealing with infected linen and waste should be followed. Feeding equipment may be cleaned and immersed in a sodium hypochlorite solution 1 in 80 for at least 30 minutes, or placed in an appropriate bag to be autoclaved. The cubicle should be cleaned daily using equipment kept for that room only. The instructions for barrier nursing should be displayed outside the cubicle, to be followed by cleaner, consultant, visitor and all.

ADMINISTRATION OF DRUGS

Special care is required when administering drugs to children. Identifying the child, calculating the dose and persuading the child to take the medicine can all cause difficulty on occasion.

The dose of a drug for a child is a fraction of the adult dose and is usually calculated according to the child's weight or some times according to his surface area. The doctor prescribes the dose and the nurse calculates how much of the stock solution is required for that dose. This can be tricky, for most drug solutions are only made up in adult doses. The calculation must be correct, errors may be fatal. Two nurses should work it out separately on paper, then compare results. If they do not agree, they both check their own calculation or get a third party to help. A junior nurse should never hesitate to say that she is not certain about the calculation — even ward sisters can make mistakes sometimes. Methods of calculation are explained at the end of this section.

It is standard practice for two nurses, one of whom is qualified, to give medicines to children. Both nurses observe the pouring out of the medicine and witness it being taken. Accurate measuring of any liquid medicine for a child is as important as the calculation, because the amounts are often small. A 5 ml plastic measure graduated in single millilitres, a 1 or 2 ml syringe or a dropper provided in some medicine bottles may all be used for measuring small amounts. The dose may then be given using a small flexible plastic measure, a spoon or in certain circumstances a syringe. The child's nameband should always be checked. It is safer if at least one of the nurses knows the child well. Children have been known to change namebands, or to give wrong names just for fun, hoping for a different coloured medicine! Medicines should never be left out in the ward or in the trolley, nor should the trolley be left unattended for a second as it is full of interest for a curious child.

Giving the medicine

Contrary to many people's opinion, many children take their medicine without any problem and some even enjoy it. The child's mother is often the best person to give the medicine or the nurse with whom the child has a good relationship and therefore trusts.

- Remain calm.
- Don't anticipate difficulty—the child quickly picks up your anxiety.
- Explain what it is if he is interested—make the explanation suitable for his age.
- Be truthful but don't exaggerate it.
- Give a choice if possible—tablet or liquid; spoon, straw or cup; mother, nurse or self to give it.
- Children will often copy other children, encourage them to copy the co-operative ones!
- Always praise the child when he has taken it.
- Offer him a drink or a sweet afterwards. A sweet is not always advisable because it creates dental problems.
- Never make a promise which cannot be kept.
- If the child is reluctant to take the medicine, make a story or game of it.
- Explain that it will make him better or take the pain away (if true).
- The medicine may be given with a teaspoonful of jam or other food but not in a large volume of fluid.

Toddlers

The toddler is likely to take his medicine when he sees others doing the same. It is best if he is taken out of his cot and sits on his mother's or the nurse's knee. He may wear a bib to protect his clothes. If he is reluctant, a firm approach may persuade him to take the medicine or he can be firmly wrapped in a small blanket with his arms controlled. The medicine can then be given in small amounts by shaping his mouth and using a small flexible medicine measure or a spoon. Small amounts at a time with intervals for swallowing and breathing reduce the risk of choking. Praise and a cuddle afterwards are important.

Babies

A bib protects the clothing. When possible, medicines are given before feeds to reduce the risk of vomiting and to ensure absorption of the drug. The baby is best held on the nurse's or mother's knee. If he has to remain in his cot, his head can be raised slightly.

A spoon is usually used, held at the baby's lips and a little of the fluid allowed to run into the mouth. The baby licks or sucks the end of the spoon and any escaping medicine will be retrieved on the spoon. Most babies have their medicine in this way, but if there is a problem, with the approval of the nurse in charge, a syringe may be used. Minimal pressure should be used on the plunger and the fluid should be placed in small amounts on the baby's tongue, not too far back, in order to avoid choking. Time should be allowed for swallowing and breathing. Medicines are never mixed in babies' bottles or in large amounts of fluid, for some may be left. If necessary, mix the drug with one or two teaspoonfuls of milk or other fluid.

If a child of any age vomits immediately after his medicine, if he refuses it or if a proportion of it is lost, the nurse in charge should be informed at once. A decision will then be made about repeating the dose or omitting it.

Methods of calculating the required volume for a child's dose

Method 1 using mathematical calculation

Step 1   Calculate the volume of stock solution containing 1 unit, e.g. 1 milligram or 1 microgram. Leave as a fraction.

Step 2   Multiply this fraction by the number of milligrams or micrograms required.

Step 3   Now work out the sum.

Step 4   Check that your answer is close to what you expected it to be.

Example

The ampoule contains 20 mg in 1 ml. The dose required is 12 mg.

Step 1   There are 20 mg in 1 ml.

Therefore there is 1 mg in $\dfrac{1}{20}$ ml.

Step 2   Therefore there are 12 mg in $\dfrac{1}{20} \times 12$ ml.

Step 3 $\dfrac{12}{20} = \dfrac{3}{5}$ ml = 0.6 ml.

Step 4   0.5 ml would contain 10 mg. The answer is just a little above this, where we would expect it to be.

If it does not seem reasonable, double check and ask someone else to check it.

Method 2 using the formula

An alternative method of calculating the required volume is to use a formula based on the method set out above. It does not unfortunately eliminate the arithmetic!

$$\frac{\text{strength required}}{\text{strength available}} \times \text{volume of stock dose} = \text{volume required}$$

Using the previous example $\dfrac{12}{20} \times 1$ ml $= \dfrac{3}{5}$ ml

$$= 0.6 \text{ ml.}$$

For those who have difficulty calculating the required volume of stock solution, a more detailed explanation with examples and practice questions is given in the Appendix (p. 308).

Administration of drugs by injection

The student is unlikely to see many children having intra-muscular injections, for most drugs are now given orally or intravenously. The intramuscular route may be used for pre-operative medication and for analgesic drugs in the early postoperative period. This route is also more likely to be used for older children and adolescents, and the procedure is similar to that for adults.

Giving the injection

Two nurses always draw up and administer the drug together. It should be drawn up away from the bedside and the nurse should avoid adjusting the syringe and needle in front of the child. Even if the child seems totally unconcerned and co-operative, he may jump or react suddenly and unexpectedly. The second nurse, therefore, should be close to the child, supporting or distracting him, with a restraining hand ready, should it be needed. If restraint is necessary, the nurse should hold the child firmly but comfortably.

A suitable and truthful explanation is given. The answer to his question 'Will it hurt?' might be 'It will hurt a little but will be over very quickly', possibly giving the reason which makes it worth while. This could be 'making the pain better' when giving an analgesic; a reward may be offered if that is possible.

After the injection the nurse should comfort the child, stay with him for a few minutes and praise him for his good behaviour. He may be helped by being allowed to express his feelings about injections and he should be left with toys or an activity of his choosing.

The needle

The needle used for an intramuscular injection should be long enough to give the medication deeply into the muscle but no bigger than necessary. It therefore depends on the child's size and the amount of muscle. A size 12 needle is suitable for many children. For subcutaneous injections a size 20 needle is used.

Sites for injections

The sites used for injections are the middle outer third and the middle anterior aspect of the thigh, the upper arm and the upper outer quadrant of the buttock. The buttocks are not used for infants or young children because of the risk of damaging the sciatic nerve. The risk is increased because of the limited amount of muscle and the smaller area of the buttocks. If the child is to have a course of intramuscular injections, all suitable sites should be used in rotation and a record should be kept. The same sites on the arm and leg may be used for subcutaneous injections.

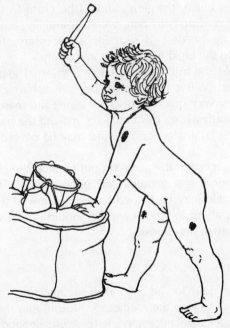

Fig. 7.2 Sites for intramuscular injections in infants and young children.

CARDIAC ARREST

One of the greatest worries for new nurses in the children's ward is the possibility of cardiac arrest occurring. Unexpected respiratory or cardiac arrest is not an everyday occurrence in the general children's ward and in many it is a rare event. It is not so different from the adult situation, for the recognition of cardiac arrest and the principles of resuscitation are similar for all age groups. Respiratory arrest is more common than cardiac arrest in children, though it inevitably leads to cardiac arrest within a few minutes if not treated promptly.

Young children are more prone to hypoxia because of their higher oxygen requirement and their lower respiratory reserve. That is why speedy action is so important when a cardiac or respiratory arrest occurs in a child. Seriously ill children and those at risk of cardiac or respiratory arrest are, whenever possible, nursed in intensive care areas. Children who are at special risk are those who have taken tricyclic antidepressant tablets such as imipramine and amitriptyline. They may have a sudden cardiac arrest several days after apparent recovery from an overdose.

During the student's first day in the ward, she should find out what the cardiac arrest procedure is for that area. This includes checking the telephone number used to call the emergency team — it may be a special number for a paediatric team. The student should find out where the emergency equipment is kept and should be familiar with the contents, noting the various sizes of laryngoscopes, airways, face masks and endotracheal tubes.

The signs of respiratory and cardiac arrest are similar to those for adults — apnoea for more than 30 seconds, pallor, greyness or cyanosis, loss of consciousness; absent heart beat, carotid or femoral pulse; dilated pupils (a late sign). Urgent medical attention is required. Do not waste time listening to the child's chest or taking his blood pressure. If a cardiac or respiratory arrest has occurred, call the emergency team at once.

Resuscitation

One nurse remains with the child, notes the time, and starts emergency treatment at once, while another nurse summons the cardiac arrest team and collects the emergency equipment. The positioning of the child, the clearing of the airway and starting mouth-to-mouth ventilation of the lungs is the same as for an adult. For smaller children, both nose and mouth can be covered by the mouth of the resuscitator. The rate of ventilation is adjusted to the normal rate of breathing, 20–40 per minute depending on the age. When equipment is available, suction can be used to clear the airway, an oral airway is inserted and 100% oxygen-enriched air given via a face mask and anaesthetic bag. A number one airway is suitable for most children between the ages of 9 months and 9 years. The anaesthetic face mask is available in various sizes and there should be a good fit of mask to patient to be effective. If there is no rise and fall of the chest when inflating the lungs, check that the airway is clear and that the mask is a good fit. The re-establishment of good lung ventilation often results in a considerable improvement in the child's condition.

External cardiac compression

If after establishing adequate ventilation, the pulses cannot be felt, external cardiac compression is started. The lower third of the sternum is compressed, using the heel of one or both hands depending on the size of the child. For smaller children, proportionately less force is required and the depth of compression of the sternum (4 cm for adults) is correspondingly less. Two finger tips may be used for a baby with a supporting hand under the chest. Alternatively two or three fingers and the thumbs can be used to enclose the chest. The number of compressions per minute varies between 60 and 100 depending on the age of the child. When combined with artificial respiration, the ratio of this to external cardiac compression is 1:5. Regurgitation of stomach contents into

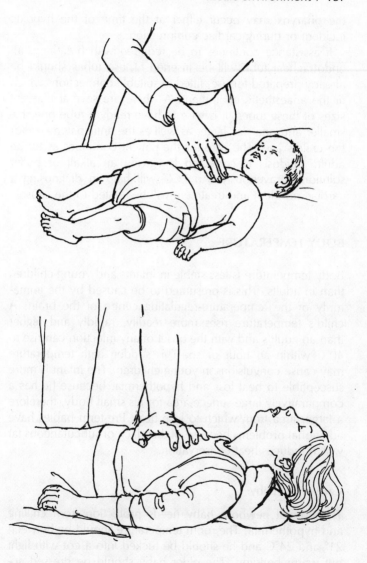

Fig. 7.3 Less force is required to carry out external cardiac compression on a child than on an adult.

the pharynx may occur either at the time of the hypoxic incident or during cardiac compression.

If assistance continues to be required with breathing, an endotracheal tube will be inserted. These tubes should be already prepared for use, fitted to suitable connections which fit the anaesthetic equipment. As there are several different sizes of these tubes, it is wise to have ready a tube one size smaller and one size larger as well as the anticipated size for the child's age. The care for the patient continues as for an adult. Acidosis is corrected by giving an alkali or buffer solution intravenously. An ECG will help in diagnosing a cardiac problem and treatment will be related to the cause.

BODY TEMPERATURE

Body temperature is less stable in infants and young children than in adults. This is presumed to be caused by the immaturity of the temperature-regulating centre of the brain. A child's temperature rises more readily, rapidly and higher than an adult's and with the onset of any infection can rise to 40°C within an hour or so. This sudden high temperature may cause convulsions in young children. The infant is more susceptible to heat loss and hypothermia, because he has a comparatively large surface area for his small body, therefore a larger area from which to lose heat. Pre-term babies have additional problems because of their lack of subcutaneous fat which reduces heat conservation.

Care of the baby

The normal newborn baby needs protection from chilling and hypothermia. The room temperature should be between 21° and 24°C and he should be tucked into a cot with light but warm bedding. The older baby should be dressed according to the environmental temperature, which is likely to be higher in hospital than at home. The baby may be warm

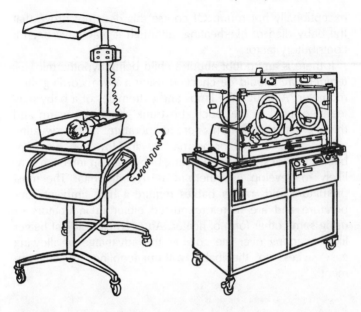

Fig. 7.4 Methods of maintaining a small baby's temperature.

enough in a vest and dress, with a little coat if he feels chilly to the touch. Bootees are usually necessary to keep his feet warm. Nylon next to the skin is uncomfortable and in hot weather, particularly, makes the babies sweat. It comes as a surprise to see a small baby in an incubator dressed in bonnet and bootees and sometimes in a dress too. Being clothed in a warm environment is better for the baby than being nursed naked in a hot one. Babies chill quickly when their clothes are removed so even in the hospital environment any examination, bathing or other procedure is carried out without any delay. If the baby is undressed for a prolonged procedure the room temperature should be raised. Overheating can also be a problem for small babies. It has been found in some instances that babies who died unexpectedly at home in their cots, had been overheated either by excessive clothing or by being left fully clothed in an exceptionally hot room. Of course this does not prove that the baby died of overheating, although it may have been a contributory factor.

If there is any doubt about a child being hypothermic, his temperature should be checked using a low-recording thermometer. Although the limbs and extremities of a baby may feel very cold to the touch, his trunk should be warm and this is a better guide to his core temperature. If he is sweating visibly he is too hot or he may be ill. However, newborn babies do not sweat and a young baby with an infection is as likely to develop *hypo*thermia as *hyper*thermia. The most premature and smaller babies require a high ambient temperature and are therefore nursed either in incubators or using some other form of heater. An overhead radiant heater like a canopy over the cot has the advantage of allowing easy access to the baby without cooling his environment.

PRACTICAL PROCEDURES

Recording the temperature

The method used to record the child's temperature depends on his age and ability to co-operate. The same site should be used each time and this should be recorded on the temperature chart. The normal temperature may vary slightly from 36.5°C to 37.2°C. It is highest when taken rectally and lowest in the axilla. Even a modest rise in temperature should be reported to the nurse in charge at once. Before the next recording the temperature may have risen to a dangerous level.

Oral temperature

The child should sit down quietly while his temperature is taken. Sensible children who are 5 years old or more may have their temperatures taken orally. This site is not used if the child has recently had a convulsion, has a history of fits, is mentally retarded or unwilling to co-operate. The thermometer is placed under his tongue and he is asked to close his lips without biting. After 2 minutes it is removed and read. If it is surprisingly low, check that the child has not just had a cold drink or an iced lollipop! Similarly a raised temperature might be due to a hot drink. Electronic temperature measuring equipment may be used; the plastic probe, which is covered by a disposable cover for each child, has the advantage of being unbreakable. It also gives an almost immediate reading. The nurse should remain near the child throughout the procedure.

Axillary temperature

This method is mostly used for children under 5 years, although in some centres it is used for all children. The nurse should remain with the young child throughout this procedure. The thermometer must be placed between the two dry surfaces of the axilla ensuring no clothing is touching the

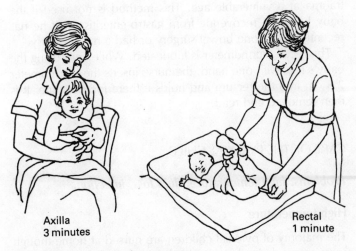

Axilla
3 minutes

Rectal
1 minute

Fig. 7.5 Recording the child's temperature.

thermometer bulb. The temperature of the child's vest is not required and may be dangerously misleading! A co-operative child will hold his arm across his chest to keep the thermometer in position. The nurse needs to check that this is maintained. It is often easier to sit a younger or less co-operative child on one's knee and hold the thermometer in position. This also provides an opportunity for contact with the child and time for a chat. The thermometer should remain in the axilla for 3 minutes, although 8 minutes is recommended for absolute accuracy. However this is considered unrealistic in practice and 3 minutes is thought to be a satisfactory compromise.

Rectal temperature

The baby's temperature is usually taken rectally. This is the most accurate of the three methods; the disadvantages are the possibility of damaging the bowel wall or the thermometer breaking if the baby kicks. Both these occurrences are very rare. An added disadvantage, if used for the toddler, is the insult of the procedure and possible psychological trauma at a vulnerable age. This method is not used if the baby has or is recovering from gastro-enteritis, or if he has recently undergone bowel surgery or had a rectal biopsy.

The rectal thermometer is lubricated. While controlling the baby's legs with one hand, the nurse inserts the thermometer 2.5 cm into the rectum and holds it there for 1 minute. It is then removed and read.

CARE OF THE PYREXIAL CHILD

Problems: high temperature, fluid loss, infection.

High temperature

The majority of pyrexial children are nursed at home though some are admitted to hospital with pyrexia of unknown origin or febrile convulsions. The child should be in a cool airy environment. A small child's clothing may be removed or he can be left in pants or a nappy if he objects to being naked. If he wants to lie down and be covered up, a cotton sheet may be used. The older child should also wear the minimum of clothing. Face and hands can be sponged frequently with tepid water which is cool and comforting. A fan may be used to cool the air but it should not blow directly onto the child, for this can cause corneal irritation. It may also constrict superficial blood vessels of the skin resulting in shivering which would warm the child up! Remember also that an electric fan is a hazard for young children and should therefore be placed at a safe distance from the pyrexial child and other children should not be allowed near it.

Paracetamol in liquid form is given orally to reduce the temperature. This may be prescribed regularly or given as necessary when the temperature is high. The child's axillary temperature is recorded half hourly or hourly, if it is very high, otherwise 4 hourly.

Fluid loss

The child is hot and sweating and needs plenty of fluids. This is not a problem unless he has a sore throat, because the child is usually thirsty. A small child may be reluctant to drink and a variety of methods and fluids can be used. If there is any doubt about how much the child is drinking, a fluid intake chart should be recorded to check the daily total.

Infection

The child is examined for signs of infection. Nose and throat swabs and a specimin of urine for culture and sensitivity will usually be taken. The commonest finding is an ear or throat infection and oral antibiotics are usually prescribed and continued for 5 days. After about 2 days of treatment the child is usually much improved and can be discharged from hospital to complete the course of antibiotics at home. Occasionally the child develops measles which only becomes apparent when the rash appears, his temperature falls and he starts to feel better.

FEBRILE CONVULSIONS

These attacks take the form of convulsive movements, like the clonic stage of a fit. The child is unconscious during the attack which may last from 1 to 20 minutes, though most are over in a few minutes. They may be called fits but they are not epileptic fits. A high temperature causes convulsions in approximately 4% of children under 5 years of age, most commonly in the second year of life. The level of temperature at which a convulsion occurs is different for each individual. In some families there is a history of parents or siblings having convulsions at the same age. Parents of a child who has had a convulsion are often very shocked and frightened and may think he is dying. They need help, an explanation and reassurance.

CARE OF THE CHILD WITH A FEBRILE CONVULSION

Problems: risk of airway obstruction, risk of physical injury, controlling the convulsion, high temperature, anxious parents, educating the parents in prevention.

Maintaining a clear airway and preventing injury

The child should be placed in the head down position or flat with his head on one side, any tight clothing round his neck and chest should be loosened. He should be protected from any surrounding danger such as sharp edges of furniture and placed in a cool environment. No attempt should be made

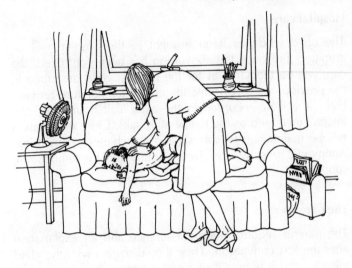

Fig. 7.6 Care of the child during a febrile convulsion at home.

to place anything between the child's teeth which are tightly clenched. This only results in damaged teeth or adults with injured fingers. In hospital, suction and oxygen should be brought to the bedside, a nurse should remain with the child while another nurse summons help.

Controlling the convulsion

Intravenous anticonvulsant drugs are given at once; one dose usually stops the fit though it will be repeated if necessary. If the convulsion is prolonged and occurs at home, the doctor should be called urgently or the child taken to hospital at once. If no transport is available, a 999 telephone call can be made for an ambulance. The child should be seen by a doctor afterwards so that any infection can be identified and treated. There is also a risk of the child having another convulsion while the temperature remains high.

Hospital care

The child who has been brought to the hospital will be admitted and once the convulsion has been controlled, the care will be the same as for the pyrexial child described in the previous section. While the child's temperature remains high, it will be recorded in the axilla half hourly and the interval increased as the temperature falls. Close observation will be maintained for any signs of twitching or convulsing. Antipyretic drugs will be given 4 hourly until the temperature subsides.

The parents

The parents require much reassurance and an explanation after the first convulsion. They should remain with the child initially, and it is best if one of the parents can be resident with him in hospital. This is better for the child and also enables the mother to participate in the child's care.

Before discharge the parents should be warned that the child may have further convulsions when his temperature rises and they should be given verbal and written instructions on how to lower his body temperature by cooling measures and giving the child paracetamol. The mother will probably have learnt this while caring for her child. The parents should also be instructed on the child's care during a convulsion. When these are difficult to control, the parents may be given a supply of diazepam and taught how to give it rectally should a convulsion occur.

The parents are reassured by the doctor that the child has not suffered any brain damage and that he is unlikely to develop epilepsy, which they often query.

BREATHING

Respiratory infections are the commonest reason for children visiting their family doctor, on average 7 times per year for children under 8 years. Although the vast majority do not require hospital care, infants and young children do develop problems more often, because of the small size of their lungs and particularly the small diameter of the air passages. Young children are also more susceptible to infection, for immunity is built up slowly from birth in response to infection.

The infant's breathing is abdominal and sometimes irregular. He breathes faster than an adult because of his high metabolic rate. Infants under 3 months are obligatory nose breathers and therefore have difficulty in breathing and feeding when their nasal passages are congested. Nasal decongestant drops may help these infants before feeds, and although feeding may be slower than usual, it is important to maintain their fluid intake.

ASSESSMENT AND IDENTIFICATION OF PROBLEMS

Assessment of the child with a respiratory infection and identifying his problems requires detailed observation both of physical signs and of the child's behaviour at a time when he is feeling least co-operative. Another difficulty in assessing the young child's condition is his inability to explain how he feels. Is the baby restless because he has cerebral hypoxia or because his napkin needs changing? Further observation and investigation may be required before the problem can be identified.

Respiratory rate

The rapid rate of respiration in the newborn period gradually slows down throughout childhood as shown in the following figures:

Age	Respiratory rate/minute
newborn	30–60
6 months	30–45
1–2 years	25–35
3–6 years	20–30
7 years +	20–25

The respiratory rate is counted for 1 minute and if the child is restless or crying the observation should be postponed until he has settled. An alternative method is to count the respirations in two 30 second periods and then add the two figures together, although this is not ideal if respiration is abnormal.

A toddler rarely co-operates for long, so if he is not having a rest or sitting quietly, he may sit on the nurse's knee and be entertained while his temperature is recorded at the same time. Older children should sit down quietly and respirations can be observed while the temperature and pulse are being taken, so that the child is unaware that he is being watched.

The infant

A convenient time for observing the infant's respirations is before he is woken for a feed, and respirations are best counted before the temperature and pulse are taken. The baby's respirations can be counted by watching the rise and fall of the chest but this is difficult when the rate is 50 or more per minute. It is easier and more accurate if the chest movement is felt by a hand placed on the infant's chest on top of his clothes.

Apnoeic attacks

Pre-term infants, and occasionally older ones too, have episodes when their breathing slows down and may stop.

These are defined as apnoeic attacks if they last for 15 seconds or longer, and they may also occur if the infant aspirates a small amount of feed. To minimise this risk, the small infant is always placed prone or on his side in the cot. Young infants with whooping cough do not whoop but may have apnoeic attacks. Apnoeic infants can often be stimulated to breathe by flicking the toes or blowing cold oxygen on the nose.

Appearance

There are many clues to the child's respiratory state in his appearance. The child may be breathless, or irritable and restless due to hypoxia. He may be pale, flushed or cyanosed. Peripheral cyanosis of hands and feet with circumoral pallor may be caused by shock or cold. On the other hand, central cyanosis in the mucous membrane of the mouth and conjunctiva is due to cardiac or respiratory disorder.

Rapid and shallow breathing occurs with pleuritic pain which accompanies lobar pneumonia or appendicitis, which sometimes mimics it. Rapid deep breathing (hyperventilation) is most commonly seen in diabetic children with keto-acidosis. The movement of the chest should be without obvious effort and equal on both sides. When breathing out is difficult and air is trapped in the lungs, as in asthma or bronchiolitis, the chest becomes over-inflated and barrel-shaped. The child's position may indicate severe dyspnoea.

Difficulty in breathing (dyspnoea)

The dyspnoeic infant is likely to be breathing approximately 50 to 70 times per minute. Respiratory distress in infants is also evident with each inspiration, in the indrawing or recession of the soft tissues of the chest wall, that is of the intercostal spaces, and above and below the sternum. This is often called chest recession or retraction.

Flaring of the nostrils may be observed in dyspnoiec children, as the accessory muscles of respiration, the alae nasi, come into play in an effort to improve oxygen intake. The child may lean forward or throw his head back on the pillow and is best left in the position which he finds most comfortable.

Respiratory noises

Snuffling, gurgling and snoring are familiar noises to all parents when their children have colds. Infection involving the pharynx and larynx causes partial obstruction of the small child's airway which results in a harsh noise on inspiration. This is called a *stridor* which is better known to mothers as *croup*. The inspiratory 'whoop' of whooping cough is quite different and follows a severe paroxysm of coughing. In contrast children with lower airway obstruction, for example bronchiolitis or asthma, *wheeze* on expiration as their problem is breathing out. They may also have an expiratory grunt as they attempt to push more air out.

Cough and sputum

A dry irritating cough which occurs with infection is troublesome and exhausting. It is of no benefit and may be suppressed by giving cough linctus. A productive cough, caused by abnormal secretions or fluids in the lower respiratory tract, helps to clear the lungs and should be encouraged. Physiotherapy may be given to encourage coughing and expectorating.

Young children are unable to expectorate, and swallow their sputum instead. If it is essential to obtain a specimen, a pharyngeal specimen may be obtained using suction. Older children providing a sputum specimen may need help, for many fail to understand the difference between saliva and sputum.

Signs of respiratory failure

The child with a respiratory problem should be constantly observed for signs of deterioration. Increasing irritability and unresponsiveness indicate hypoxia of the brain. Other signs are a rising pulse rate, cyanosis and increasing respiratory effort. These signs may develop slowly, but they may also occur suddenly without warning, and the child may require immediate nasotracheal intubation and assisted ventilation. The asthmatic child who stops wheezing, but continues to have other serious signs, is probably too weak to breathe adequately, and equally requires urgent attention.

PRACTICAL PROCEDURES

Taking a throat and nose swab

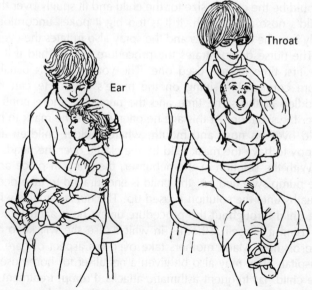

Fig. 7.7 Holding the child for throat examination or taking a swab, and for ear examination.

Assistance is required from his mother or a nurse to hold a young child firmly while a throat swab is taken. The infant is most easily restrained in a small blanket wrapped firmly round him. A good light is required and a spatula to keep the tongue down. If the child can co-operate, ask him to say 'Ahhh' and the spatula may not be needed. The swab must not touch any part of the mouth or teeth, and if this happens a new swab should be used. Similarly a nose swab must be inserted into the nostril and not wiped round the opening.

Administration of drug by nebuliser

The child with an asthmatic attack is often treated with bronchodilator drugs which are most effective when given by inhalation using an electric compressed air pump or nebuliser. $\frac{1}{2}$ to 1 ml of salbutamol is added to 1 to 2 ml of water or normal saline and given over 5 to 10 minutes. The mask should be the correct size for the child and fit snugly over the child's nose and mouth. If it is too big it pokes uncomfortably into the child's eyes and the spray also irritates the eyes.

The nurse demonstrates the procedure to the child if it is the first time he has used one. The young child is usually more comfortable sitting on the nurse's knee. He can be cuddled at the same time and the nurse has more control over the situation. At this age he often prefers the mask to be held over his nose and mouth, whereas older children are happy to have the mask held by the elastic over the head.

With the solution in the nebuliser, the mask in place and the pump switched on, the child is encouraged to take deep breaths until the solution is used up. The nurse remains with the child throughout the procedure unless he is accustomed to using it himself at home, in which case she will keep an eye on him. Many mothers take over this aspect of care in hospital. They may also be given a nebuliser for home use if the child has frequent asthmatic attacks. Prompt treatment is often effective in reducing the severity of the attacks and cuts down the number of hospital admissions.

Administration of oxygen

Oxygen may be given to children by oxygen tent, mask, nasal catheters, incubator, head box or Derbyshire chair. The latter is a baby chair fitted with an oxygen attachment and a transparent hood over the baby's head. The oxygen tent is used here as an example.

Oxygen therapy can be frightening for a child so an explanation beforehand is essential. If it is a planned procedure and not an emergency, the child can be prepared earlier.

Some tents have containers for ice and water to keep the tent cool and to humidify the air. Others are electrically controlled.

Preparation and commencing therapy

- Explain to the child and parents about the tent and what is to happen if not already done.
- Ensure that the mattress has a plastic cover. If not, it should be covered with a plastic sheet.
- Check that all parts are to hand and in good order, particularly noting that the canopy is not torn and that all connections fit well.
- Erect the tent and attach the canopy. This may be a matter of trial and error the first time. If possible, practise in a quiet moment before it is needed in an emergency.
- Place ice in the ice box, fill the humidifier with distilled water or set the controls.
- Flush the tent through with oxygen for 5 minutes before placing the child in it.
- Make the child comfortable and ensure that pillows or other objects are not obstructing the oxygen inlets.
- Tuck the canopy in carefully all around the mattress to prevent oxygen, which is heavier than air, from escaping.
- Make sure that all openings are securely closed.

- Give the child some toys; avoid electric or sparking ones.
- Encourage the mother to stay. Help her to care for the child if she wishes and if it is possible.
- If she cannot stay, remain with the child until he settles down.

Observations during oxygen therapy

The child

- Look at the child at least every quarter of an hour.
- Observe all respiratory signs and record with pulse rate regularly, for example hourly.
- Record the child's axillary temperature frequently if it is fluctuating.
- Check if bedding or clothing is damp and change as necessary.

The equipment

- Maintain tent temperature at 18–21°C (65–70°F) and record hourly.
- Measure oxygen concentration in the tent hourly using an oxygen analyser.
- Check the connections frequently and the level of ice and water from time to time. Check oxygen cylinders similarly, if used.

Nursing or medical attention and observations which disturb the child should, where possible, be timed to coincide, in order to allow the child maximum rest.

Safety precautions

Fire precautions should be taken, visitors should be warned and a notice should be displayed on the tent. Special care is required in the children's ward where there are always many visitors nearby who may be unaware of the risks. There should be no smoking, lighting of matches, nor electrical equipment or toys in the vicinity which might cause a spark. No oil should be used on equipment.

CARE OF THE BABY WITH BRONCHIOLITIS WHO IS BREATHLESS

Many dyspnoeic babies, suffering from bronchiolitis, are admitted to paediatric wards each winter. This infection is usually caused by the respiratory syncytial virus (RSV) and is most serious in infancy. The small bronchioles and bronchi become narrowed and sometimes obstructed by inflammation and sticky secretions. As a result, breathing out is particularly difficult—air is trapped in the alveoli and the lungs become over-inflated causing the chest to become barrel-shaped. Small babies and those who are severely affected require hospital care.

Bronchiolitis begins with coryza followed by an irritable cough and difficulty in breathing and feeding. In severe cases the baby has a respiratory rate of 50–70 per minute and extreme dyspnoea. He is unable to feed normally and may be cyanosed.

Problems: difficulty in breathing, coughing, restlessness and exhaustion, reduced fluid intake, risk of dehydration and anxious parents.

Difficulty in breathing

The baby is admitted into a warm room where oxygen and suction are available. His mother is welcomed and asked to remain with the baby, if she can, to comfort him. The baby should be handled as little as possible but an accurate weight is essential. As well as being used for calculating fluid requirement and drug dosage, a rapid weight increase is a sign of heart failure which occasionally develops. While he is being weighed, a quick assessment of his responsiveness, colour, chest movement and rate of respiration can be made.

The baby is placed in a baby chair to aid breathing. Care should be taken to ensure that the chair is stable and that the restraining straps around the waist and between the legs are always fastened. The baby is in the best position when lying back slightly, to prevent him falling forwards and hampering his breathing. An alternative to a chair is a slanting board placed underneath the mattress, or pillows under the head end of the mattress to raise it. A small baby can be supported on the incline by placing a rolled-up napkin under the buttocks. The cotsides should be fully raised when the baby is unattended in a baby chair or lying on an inclined board.

Oxygen which is always humidified is given if the baby is cyanosed or severely dyspnoeic. The guidelines already described should be followed. Maintaining the correct concentration of oxygen is important and blood gas levels of the seriously ill baby may be measured so that the correct amount is given. Oxygen therapy of pre-term (premature) babies is always monitored in this way, because high arterial concentrations of oxygen may cause blindness (retrolential fibroplasia) in this special group.

Gentle nasopharyngeal suction is sometimes used to remove secretions from the baby's mouth and pharynx but this should not be carried out without instructions except in an emergency, for over-enthusiastic use of suction may cause irritation and increase the secretions.

The baby is constantly observed with frequent recordings of respiration and pulse rate. He is also closely watched for signs of deterioration such as increased chest wall recession, worsening colour and restlessness.

Restlessness and exhaustion

After the baby has been examined and weighed and essential observations recorded, he is dressed in light, easily removed clothing which does not hamper his breathing and permits easy observation of his chest movement. He should have the maximum amount of rest, with his care co-ordinated to avoid unnecessary disturbance. Initially daily bathing may be omitted but the baby's face, hands and skin creases should be kept clean. Particular attention should be given to the napkin area to prevent any soreness resulting from the baby's position. A slight adjustment to his position 2 hourly is beneficial. The baby may require yellow paraffin on his lips; if he is well hydrated, special mouth care is not required.

Reduced fluid intake and risk of dehydration

The baby with a rapid respiratory rate cannot breathe and suck at the same time. He has probably not been able to take all his feeds and may have been vomiting. He is therefore often dehydrated.

The normal fluid intake must be maintained although the older baby's weaning diet is discontinued temporarily. Dyspnoeic babies are fed by nasogastric tube because they have difficulty feeding, they are exhausted by the effort of breathing and they are unable to take the amount of milk they need. Severely dyspnoeic babies may be given half the normal 4 hourly feed 2 hourly by tube, and if this is not tolerated, clear fluids may be given instead, for 24 hours. During the tube feed, the nurse should watch for signs of intolerance such as retching, restlessness, or a deterioration in colour. The baby may vomit or develop abdominal distension and if any of these occur, the feed should be stopped and advice sought.

When the baby's condition starts to improve after a few days, he is able to start sucking again. Initially he may tire before he has finished a feed so the remainder can be given by tube. The baby's cough, which may persist for some time, is troublesome and may prolong the feed. By the time he is discharged he should be feeding normally and gaining weight.

Anxious parents

Most parents are anxious when their child is ill, but more so when he is unable to breathe properly. They are made welcome and one of them is encouraged to stay with the baby. Details of the condition are discussed with them so that they may be partly reassured by understanding the treatment and the usual course of the condition. They are also encouraged to ask questions. When the baby is settled and the parents are more relaxed, the nursing history is taken.

Parents are encouraged to help with the baby's care, even if initially this is just by holding his hand. As soon as possible, his mother is encouraged to take over his care. The baby's cough may persist for a while, but if he is improving and his mother is managing the feeding, the baby may be discharged home.

CROUP

This is another condition seen in young children. Laryngo-tracheobronchitis or croup is a viral infection in which the small child develops an inspiratory stridor due to inflammation and narrowing of his comparatively narrow larynx.

Typically, a toddler who has a cold, wakes during the night with a harsh inspiratory stridor which frightens him and his parents. Most children can be cared for at home. The child is comforted on his parent's knee, given a warm drink and propped up in his cot. Mothers find that a steamy atmosphere or patent vaporiser in the room often relieves the symptoms.

The child is admitted to hospital with a severe attack or if his condition is deteriorating, for he then requires close observation. Humidified oxygen using a tent may be given and oxygen is essential if the child is cyanosed or severely dyspnoeic. A calm confident approach, rest and plenty of fluids are required.

Taking a throat swab, passing a nasogastric tube and pharyngeal suction must not be carried out, for irritation of the inflamed layrnx may precipitate complete obstruction and a respiratory arrest. Very occasionally nasotracheal intubation is required to maintain the child's airway.

REFERENCES AND FURTHER READING

Infection (Part I) Nursing 2 (7): 1982 November
Infection (Part II) Nursing 2 (8): 1982 December

Communicating
  The infant
  The toddler and pre-
    school child
  The deaf or hearing-
    impaired child
  The visually-
    handicapped child
  The child in pain

Playing
  Functions of play
  Play and toys related
    to age
  Play in hospital
  Play and treatment
School
  Hospital school

8

Communicating, playing, school

COMMUNICATING

Language and intellectual development go hand in hand, for understanding precedes expression at most ages. The 1-year-old is a good example, for he understands simple commands but only says 2 or 3 words.

THE INFANT

The newborn infant's communication with the world is largely non-verbal through his mother's touch and handling, and his response to her. As she talks to him, he learns the melody and tone of language, so that by 6 months he can differentiate between anger and pleasure in her voice. The baby also talks in his own way from birth. It is easy to differentiate between the distressed cry of the young baby and his contented gurgling and cooing when he has been fed.

During the first year the baby's sounds turn into babbling, strings of sounds without any resemblance to speech. This is followed by scribble talk which sounds like distant conversation. By 12 to 15 months recognisable words are used as labels, each having many meanings and sometimes acting as one word sentences.

THE TODDLER AND PRE-SCHOOL CHILD

As vocabulary and understanding increase, the child talks in telegraphic style, in 2 to 3 word sentences. By the age of 3½ to 4 years many children have a good grasp of grammar although pronunciation may not conform to the adult form. At each stage the child's speech is appropriate and correct for his age.

Delayed language development

Language development may be delayed because of social factors, lack of conversation or lack of encouragement to talk in the home. It may also occur if the child's hearing is impaired, or because he is physically handicapped or has cerebral damage. A structural defect, such as a cleft palate, may affect speech. Stammering is quite common in children under 4 years and is best ignored. The child should not be asked to repeat the words. Neither should he be told to speak more slowly nor to think about what he is saying.

THE DEAF OR HEARING-IMPAIRED CHILD

Loss of hearing may be congenital or the result of a head injury, a serious infection such as meningitis, or ear infections. The child may be partially deaf, severely deaf or profoundly deaf, and in each group, different problems affect how the child communicates and the help he requires.

The partially deaf child hears normal speech close to, but not a quiet voice. He omits many of the quiet consonants from the beginning and end of words, for example he says 'up' for 'cup'. He should learn to use a hearing aid quite easily and with it he will be able to hear normal speech.

The severely deaf child does not hear speech without a hearing aid but will react to a loud shout at close range. With his aid he is more aware of everyday sounds in the room. He will hear the rhythm and sounds of speech but not distinctly. With a lot of practice he will be able to differentiate between similar sounding words in quiet surroundings. However, many consonants will still be distorted or barely heard though this can be overcome in time. In noisy situations he will not hear clearly and will have to lip read at times.

The profoundly deaf child without a hearing aid only reacts to the vibration of heavy banging or similar noise. With an aid set at maximum he is aware of traffic noise and in a quiet room can hear the rhythm of the voice. He is dependent on lip reading for most communication.

Helping the child with impaired hearing

Because the child does not hear his own voice normally, his speech may be softer or louder than usual. This should be corrected by gentle reminders otherwise the child will lose confidence in talking, and speech may regress. Behaviour problems may occur because the child's impaired hearing makes him less aware of other people's needs and he is more likely to be introverted. His language development has also probably been slowed up so that he may be inclined to resort to tears and gestures although his intelligence is normal.

The adult can help the child by remaining calm and finding out the child's problem. A solution can then be found or the child told firmly that what he wants is not allowed. The adult's facial expression and simple comments of praise or disapproval are soon understood by the child, if the same words are used consistently in similar situations. A partially deaf child and some severely deaf ones who are using a hearing aid, will understand the tone of voice even if not the words. The child must understand why he is being punished or praised. He should also understand what is expected of him. Punishment without understanding creates resentment and more problems for him.

The deaf child is only handicapped by defective hearing but if he is pampered and special allowances made for him, he is given an additional handicap. The child needs help to remain normal and under no circumstances should he be pitied.

The child with a hearing aid

The deaf child with a hearing aid hears best if the speaker talks at normal loudness about 4 feet away from him. Too loud a voice or being too close to the microphone distorts the speech and a quiet voice cannot be heard. The nearer you are to the aid, the quieter your voice should be and the further away you are, the louder it should become. The greater the distance between the speaker and the aid, the less distinct the speech becomes, because the aid picks up all the noises in between.

When speaking to a deaf person with or without an aid, avoid overemphasising words or breaking up sentences which upsets the rhythm of speech and makes it more difficult for the deaf person to understand. Hearing aids should be maintained in good condition and positioned correctly in the ear.

The deaf child in hospital

The deaf child is naturally more apprehensive than a child with normal hearing when he is admitted to hospital. The young child benefits if his mother is resident and older children, too, benefit from a parent staying for the first few days.

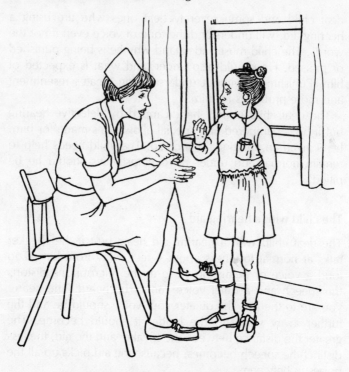

Speak clearly and a little more slowly than usual.
Don't over-exaggerate lip movements.
Don't hide your mouth with your hand.

Fig. 8.1 Always face a deaf child when talking to him, and make sure that your face is in a good light.

The initial contact is important, welcoming the child by talking and relating to him directly as well as using facial expression and gestures. Having his own nurse will help him and information about how he normally communicates should be written in the nursing record. This might be, for example, 'lip reading only' or 'limited hearing plus lip reading', as well as other means of communication such as sign language. Sign language cards which give the signs and their meanings can be obtained. Details about the hearing aid and its use are also required. Is it worn continuously, how is it worn and can the child manage it himself? Spare batteries should be available.

The child should be nursed in an area with other children, he should be introduced to them and they should all be encouraged to play together. All staff in the area should be aware of the child's handicap and a note to this effect should be written on or attached to the front of his notes. Explanations require thought and initiative, and demonstrations and drawings will be easier for the child to understand than a complicated explanation. Prior to surgery, the hearing aid should be left in position until the child has been anaesthetised.

THE VISUALLY-HANDICAPPED CHILD

Visually-handicapped children are admitted to the paediatric ward with the same disorders as normally sighted children, for example appendicitis. A child may have a squint corrected or be admitted with an eye injury but most children with eye disorders are treated in special ophthalmic units. Children whose treatment necessitates covering the eyes should be considered as 'blind' during this period.

Many children who are registered as blind, have limited sight so the nurse should first find out how much the child can see. He may have no vision on one side or beyond 3 feet. His central vision may be affected or he may have difficulty in focusing.

Care of the visually-handicapped child in hospital

Children who have adjusted to their visual handicap are usually determinedly independent and this should be encouraged in hospital. The child should be shown his bed and the immediate area by feeling around it and using what sight he has. He should arrange his own belongings in his locker so that he knows where he can find them. He should be taken round the ward and any hazards or objects which appear hazy to him should be explained. Lighting may need adjusting, for some partially sighted children see better in a bright light but others require shaded light. When watching television the child should be placed in the position which suits him best.

The child can choose his own toys and should be encouraged to join in activities with other children who need to be told about the blind child's handicap. Large print books and tape recorders are useful but should not replace the company of adults or other children. The young child needs toys of different textures, shapes and sizes. Those which make a noise are helpful and ones which move encourage him to explore his environment.

Talking to the visually-handicapped

The child should be approached from the side of 'best vision' to prevent him being taken by surprise. A warning of approach such as 'Hello Robert, this is Nurse Black' avoids startling the child, tells him that he is being addressed and also who the speaker is and how far away he is. His name should be said first for, when others are present, it is the only way he can tell that he is being spoken to. The nurse should always speak before touching him and explain what she is going to do before starting.

At mealtimes the food on the plate should be described and he should be told where it is on the plate. When walking with a blind child, give him the choice of how he is helped. He should never be pushed or hurried and can be guided by the arm. Clear instructions about direction and hazards ahead should be given.

THE CHILD IN PAIN

The statement 'pain is whatever the experiencing person says it is' (McCaffery, 1979) is true for all ages except young children who cannot say what it is, and may in fact confuse the situation trying to explain. A 3-year-old is quite likely to say that he has tummy ache when he has a sore throat. The distress of the child who is too young to communicate can only be presumed from the sound of his cry, and by observing his behaviour and reactions to a situation.

The meaning of pain

A child's pain is not necessarily physical, and most adults would probably agree that a feeling of unhappiness or distress is part of pain. For the young child, pain is likely to mean separation from his mother; the school-age child may interpret pain as a punishment and therefore fear rejection. Pain may be associated with guilt or be interwoven with ideas of death or fear of the unknown. A physical symptom, such as pain, may also be a response to emotional stress at home or at school.

The child's reaction to pain

This depends partly on the child's age and his cultural and family background. Children's reactions to pain reflect the attitude of those around them and they therefore respond much as their parents do. Some ignore a grazed knee while others need comfort and a plaster. They may respond differently in front of their peers at school or in hospital, wanting to appear brave.

Previous experiences may affect the child's reaction to pain. For example a 9-year-old, who had suffered severe attacks of tonsillitis, complained less than the other children after tonsillectomy. When asked about his sore throat postoperatively he said that it was not very painful and much less so than during attacks of tonsillitis.

Perception of pain and discomfort may be increased by fear, stress, boredom, depression and anticipation of pain. Children may have all of these feelings.

Identifying the child in pain

The older child may tell the nurse that he is in pain, although many dislike admitting it and try to avoid showing it. They would rather suffer than have an injection to relieve it. Another child who looks flushed or tense might be relieved to admit to pain, when asked directly during a quiet chat.

The pre-school child will try to explain his pain, which alerts the staff to something being wrong, though the words he uses may be incorrect. 'A sore tummy' probably means that something is hurting somewhere in the body. Pointing to the area of the body with one finger may be helpful but again it can be misleading.

Babies and young children who are unable to talk, and sometimes older ones too, show by changes in their behaviour that something is wrong. The child may be unsettled or adopt an unusual posture, or the baby may refuse his feed or never settle for long. Knowing the child's normal behaviour helps the nurse to identify signs of pain and for the same reason the parents may be the first people to realise that something is wrong.

Assessing the severity of pain

The nurse needs to listen to the child and his family. She needs to observe the child's facial expression, as well as noting any aggression, irritability, inactivity or withdrawal. Those with chronic pain may be depressed but uncomplaining. Other signs may be a raised pulse or respiratory rate, an alteration in skin colour or sweating.

Important questions to ask are:

- Does the pain interrupt sleep or play?
- Does the pain destroy appetite?
- Does the pain make the child cry?
- Does the pain make the older child want to cry even if he is not actually crying?

When a child has an obvious cause for pain, other secondary causes should not be forgotten. Conditions, such as cystitis or constipation, can cause acute discomfort and pain, and may be overlooked.

Relieving the child's pain

There are several ways of helping to relieve children's pain including the administration of analgesics which are often under-used.

Discomfort and pain may be alleviated by basic nursing measures such as changing the child's position, making him comfortable, re-arranging pillows, or where appropriate, rubbing the injured part or adjusting splints, tubes, or dressings. Local application of heat, safely applied, can be soothing.

Drugs are used if simple measures are not effective or when pain is severe. The aim is to control and therefore prevent pain rather than to relieve it, so that the fear of pain with its resulting tension is removed. When analgesics are required regularly, they should be given promptly and before the child complains. In this way, pain is usually controlled by less analgesic. The more pain is experienced, the lower the patient's tolerance becomes. Whenever possible, children are given oral analgesics.

General anaesthetics are often used for children undergoing unpleasant procedures which adults have to tolerate. It may be the only method of keeping the child still, but it is also to avoid the trauma and pain of the procedure. Older children with leukaemia, who have regular bone marrow punctures and lumbar punctures, may be offered a general

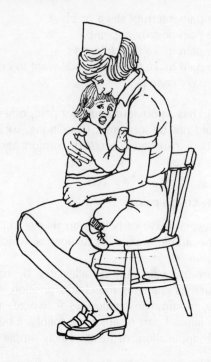

Fig. 8.2 Physical contact is often the best way to comfort a child.

anaesthetic or an intravenous injection and they choose which they will have.

When a child complains of pain unexpectedly and no physical cause is found, it is worth finding out if anything is worrying him. Fears or uncertainties may be the cause or at least a contributory factor. Explanation, discussion and telling someone may sometimes solve the problem. The child can often be distracted and forget his pain if he becomes absorbed in a game, and play may help him to act out his fears and therefore reduce tension. Being rocked or cuddled by a familiar person often helps babies and children to quieten and relax. If the child is confined to bed, his forehead or arm can be stroked instead.

PLAYING AND SCHOOL

Play is a serious business to the child, as anyone knows who has watched children at play. Play is spontaneous and enjoyable. It provides moments of delight when the child creates something or achieves a longed-for goal. Play can also be entertaining and certainly has its humorous side. The child does not normally have to be asked to play, nor does he need help to play though this is sometimes beneficial. Having no toys does not stop him playing for he will improvise with what he finds around him.

FUNCTIONS OF PLAY

The child would not give the activities listed below as his reasons for playing but they are benefits which occur naturally when the child plays. Play strengthens the child's body, improves his mind, helps him to learn social skills and develops his personality. Play provides opportunities for experimenting, practising and achieving in a world of his own, where mistakes need not matter and he is without unwanted adult interference. Most of these activities involve learning in one way or another.

In play the child:
— enjoys himself
— explores his environment
— is stimulated
— satisfies curiosity
— develops his imagination
— relates to other children and learns to share
— acts out aggression, anxieties and fears
— practises adult roles
— solves his own everyday problems.

Play is a vital factor in intellectual, social and emotional development: it changes as the child develops.

Birth–1 year

The baby learns about himself and the world by movement and contact with people and objects. His mother is his most valuable plaything for the first few months of life. She is pleasant to touch and does not mind her eyes and mouth being poked by inquisitive fingers. She is responsive and understanding, providing movement and appropriate conversation. The baby needs variety in his surroundings, and as he becomes more mobile he needs space, and encouragement to move around.

Toys and activities for the infant

Toys to hold, handle and manipulate, to watch or pick up, to drop, roll or throw; toys which rattle, squeak or produce a tune, toys of different colours and textures.

Examples: mobiles and dangling toys, soft toys, rattles, teething rings, rubber bath toys which squeak, plastic rings or animals on a string or an assortment of different articles attached to a string across the cot or pram, crinkly paper, rubber or cloth blocks, squeezy toys, small wooden bricks, large plastic ball, cloth book, bouncing on adult knee to rhyme or song, hide and find games, peek-a-boo or pat-a-cake.

1–3 years

The 1-year-old practises and enjoys large movements and is learning to co-ordinate fine movements. From around 2 years the child's play becomes imitative so domestic play is common. In symbolic play the child uses an object to represent something quite different. From playing alone, the toddler starts to play alongside other children but not with them. He progresses to watching others at play and eventually joins in.

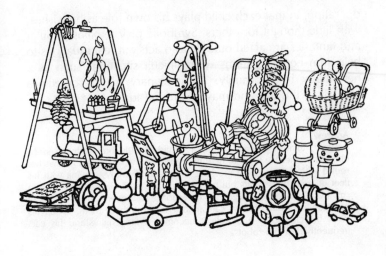

Fig. 8.3 Toys for 1- to 3-year olds.

Toys and activities for the toddler

Toys on a string to pull, or on wheels to push or pull, toys to sit astride and push along with feet; sliding or swinging (small swing), fetching and carrying, building up and knocking down, putting in and taking out, domestic play or helping in the home.

Examples: 'sit and ride' tractor or car, tricycle, climbing frame, slide, barrow, large ball; plastic or wooden trains, cars or boats; posting boxes, hammer pegs on frame, pop-up toys, plasticine or play dough, finger paints, blackboard and chalks, wooden or plastic engine or boat, wooden animal and farm set, lift-out picture board, iron, sweeping brush, cooking set, soap bubbles, large print picture books.

3–5 years

The child's movements are more controlled and better co-ordinated. Children play together but there is no true co-operation, in that each child plays his own role as he wishes, with little thought for others. Symbolic play remains popular and fantasies are acted out. He also acts out real situations to help him come to terms with difficult situations such as a new baby in the family. An imaginary friend sometimes appears at this age and may be around for years.

Andrew

Andrew, almost 4 years old, is a confident little boy with a serious outlook on life. He loves to help his mother in the house and follows her round with the sweeping brush or a duster. He enjoys playing with his fleet of small model cars but his favourite toy is his BMX bicycle; 'not a small one' he replies indignantly in response to a query about its size. It has stabilisers but Andrew can almost ride it without them. When his BMX bicycle is not a bicycle it becomes a fire engine and his cars frequently turn into robots.

Andrew's fantasy world is very real to him and he will talk to his cars as if they were robots. The 3-year-old loves to help adults with real jobs, and in doing this as well as in domestic play, Andrew is practising the adult role and finding out how it feels.

Toys and activities for the pre-school child

Toys for movement and opportunities for climbing, toys with several parts to be taken apart and put together, toys for domestic play, helping in the house, simple sorting, everyday objects for inventive play.

Examples: tricycles, bicycles, scooters, slides, tea chests, car tyres, Wendy houses, dolls' prams, cots, dressing-up clothes with props, model cars, garages, scales, painting with brush, crayons, glove puppets, cutting out, interlocking shapes, scrap books, threading beads, matching card games, telephone, simple building sets, cooking (supervised), simple woodwork (supervised).

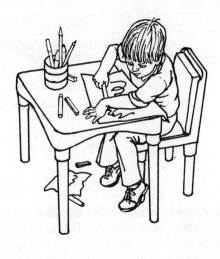

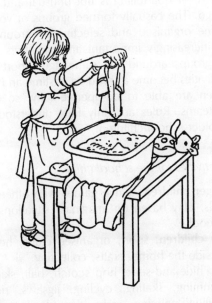

Fig. 8.4 Play activities for the pre-school child.

Table 8.1 Social play

Type of play	Age	Children's activity
Solitary	Infancy	Play independently with no interest in others
Parallel	Toddler	Play alongside others but not involved with them
Associative	Pre-school	Play with others but there is no organisation
Co-operative	School-age	Plan and discuss activities and belong to the group

5–12 years

The child now prefers to play with other children. 'Not going out to play' matters to a 5-year-old. Young children often have a special friend, or perhaps a trio play together at school. However quarrelling is not unusual and friendships come and go. The casually formed groups of younger children become organised and selective by around 8 years. Gangs are increasingly important and members divide into single sex groups around the same age. Sport and other outdoor activities become a favourite pastime and for the first time children are able to co-operate fully, so they enjoy playing in teams. Rules are only fully understood and accepted by older school children.

Toys and activities for the school child

For younger children: active games with others involving specific skills, play based on imaginary situations based on home or school.

For older children: sport, organised clubs, hobbies and interests outside the home, crafts, collecting.

Examples: hide-and-seek, hop scotch, ball, skipping in a group, swimming, skating, cycling, jigsaws, riddles and magic, drawing, painting, embroidery, basket work, dolls with accessories (male and female), reading, fishing, cycling, model making, music making or listening, television, chemistry set, gang activities; outings to leisure park, cinema or football match.

Adolescent

The adolescent relies on his group of friends for companionship and leisure pursuits. Sport, hobbies, meeting at youth clubs, and listening to music are likely pastimes.

Examples of games and activities: swimming, cycling, football, tape recorder, radio, tinkering with motor cycle, chess, dominoes, draughts, card games, board games, television, reading newspaper and magazines.

PLAY IN HOSPITAL

Play should be possible for a child whatever his age in any situation. In hospital it provides reassuring links with home. The child can play familiar games, read favourite stories or play with his own toys if he wishes. Often children prefer the novelty of the toys in the ward and the company of new friends. When the child is absorbed in an interesting activity he is more likely to forget about his own problems. Opportunities for developing and learning new skills in play are also available in hospital.

Places for play

The youngest baby should have a soft toy, a string of toys across his cot or a mobile above it. A child may play in bed, on the ward floor, in the playroom or outside. The playroom is usually more spacious and has no reminders of hospital such as medical equipment or the smell of disinfectant. Children can feel safe in the playroom when medical and nursing procedures are forbidden there. Very few play activities are impossible in bed or cot. Sand and water play can be arranged if the bedclothes are adequately protected.

Handicapped children

Physically handicapped children require help when positioning themselves for play in order to gain most from their activity. The child may be able to play on the floor in the lateral position if he is well supported. Alternatively he may be better lying prone on a wedge (Fig. 8.5) with his upper body raised so that his hands and arms are free. The child in a wheelchair should again be well supported, the play surface should be close to him and at a comfortable height. He may find it easier to sit in an ordinary chair at a table. This has the added advantage that it is a normal position and he can mix more easily with the other children.

Play for the mentally handicapped must be geared to their level of understanding and practical ability, therefore assessing the child's ability is an essential prerequisite. Usually simple toys are required which do not depend on fine manipulative skills although this may be included as part of a

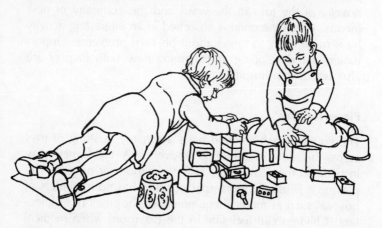

Fig. 8.5 Helping the handicapped child to play actively.

training programme. Most of these children are being trained in social skills, such as learning to dress themselves or learning to use a spoon, and play may be incorporated where it is appropriate. They enjoy music and movement in group activities and also outings for horse-riding, shopping, to the country or to the seaside.

PLAY AND TREATMENT

Play can be useful in unexpected circumstances. The seriously ill child may not have the energy to play actively or even to read a book but he may appreciate listening to a story read to him or watching an adult drawing a picture. The use of a tape recorder to stimulate unconscious patients is well known.

Mary Claire

Mary Claire, who was 13 years old, had been unconscious for 3 weeks as a result of a road traffic accident. Her condition was stable but she had remained unconscious and had not spoken since the accident. Her parents sitting at her bedside were amazed when she suddenly sat bolt upright in bed one afternoon and started to talk about her favourite television programme. Then they realised that the familiar signature tune had provided the stimulus as the programme started on the ward television.

Doctors and nurses often use play in order to gain the child's co-operation during a procedure. The child who is reluctant to have his temperature taken may be persuaded by helping to take teddy's first. The child who is frightened of the weighing scales may be reassured if a nurse or his mother is weighed too. The toddler playing with the nurse's watch while she takes his pulse may help (or hinder) her.

Explanations using play

Explanations about the child's treatment can sometimes be incorporated into a story. A child who will be in an oxygen tent postoperatively may be shown it beforehand and the nurse may tell him a story which involved his toys and the tent as a little house. A child who hated his regular blood transfusions was helped by the nurse who told him the story about Berty Bloodbag and his army of goodies helping to kill off the bad cells in his body.

An effective method of explaining to children what a plaster of Paris cast will look like is to apply an identical plaster to a doll. The child can then see it, handle it and if necessary it can be removed to show the doll's body intact underneath. This method is also useful for small children who imagine that a part of their body has disappeared.

Stephen

Stephen, an adventurous 3½-year-old, had trapped his hand in his mother's washing machine. The injury required plastic surgery and following his operation Stephen was very unhappy about his bandaged hand. He wanted his hand back and could not accept that it was there because he could not see it. His nurse spent time with him, bandaging and unbandaging teddy's paw showing how the paw always came back. Stephen enjoyed this activity and helped with his good hand. While this may not have been his only problem, he was noticeably happier after the demonstration of teddy's paw.

Stephen might have been helped more if the demonstration of teddy's paw had been given pre-operatively. Pre-operative explanations require careful thought to ensure that they are not going to frighten the child and therefore be counter productive.

Hospital play

In hospital, children quickly learn about the activities of staff and their own role as patients. It can be disconcerting and sometimes entertaining to overhear conversations and to recognise individual members of staff, either by manner or conversation, in an accurate replay of the morning's events.

The game of doctors and nurses provides a valuable outlet for children to express their fears and frustrations and 'for

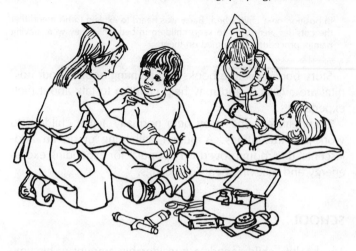

Fig. 8.6 'Is it serious?'

getting their own back' by energetically injecting dolls or removing their tonsils. Dressing-up clothes are popular and hospital equipment such as masks, stethoscopes, syringes without needles, and charts should be provided. A few patients, dolls, teddies or animals plus pieces of material which pass as blankets make it more realistic. Ideally a permanent hospital corner should be set up in the ward where the children are free to play at any time. A smaller version using a doll family and a miniature ward may be useful for bedfast children to enable them to talk about their feelings concerning hospital. During this type of play, opinions, misconceptions about hospitals and treatment are often brought into the open. Sometimes an adult needs to set up hospital play with a group though often play is spontaneous and the adult need only intervene to correct misconceptions or to make a particular point.

Barry

Barry was 5 years old when he had a minor operation which necessitated a short stay in hospital. He was a thoughtful little boy who was interested in all the ward activities. Some time after observing cotsides being placed in position on a child's bed, Barry was heard to explain to his friend that the cotsides were used to keep children in bed while they were having painful procedures performed on them.

Story books, picture books and painting books about hospital are available and may help children to talk about their experiences.

Competitive games may help normally active children to work out frustrations. A punch ball hung up in an adolescents' day room proved very popular for expending excess energy and relieving pent-up feelings.

SCHOOL

The healthy child spends a considerable amount of his time at school and involved in school activities. Many children enjoy talking about their favourite subjects and extramural activities.

The child enters school at 5 years but this varies slightly because some schools take children in the year before their 5th birthday. There are many patterns of schooling depending on the Local Education Authority, and therefore children do not all move to a more senior school at the same age.

Table 8.2 Different ages for transferring to a new school

	Age in years	
	Enter	Leave
Example 1		
Primary school	5	11
infants 5–7		
junior 8–11		
Secondary school	11	16 (minimum)
Example 2		
First school	5	8–10
Middle school	8–10	12–13
Upper school	12–13	16 (minimum)

HOSPITAL SCHOOL

Some children gleefully anticipate missing school while they are in hospital. Their enthusiasm is initially dampened when they find out that school continues in hospital for all children who are well enough to join in, however short their stay. Children recovering from serious illness may attend for short spells and be given easier work than they had previously been doing. Children in bed receive as much attention as those who can go to the ward classroom. Continuing schooling without interruption enables the child to keep up with his school work and sometimes he receives more individual help than is possible in his normal school. A full range of subjects is covered and facilities can be provided for children to take public examinations if necessary. School activities may include craft work, nature walks, outings to places of interest and musical sessions.

The child may benefit from his enjoyment of school work; it may be a challenge to him and distract him from his condition. It may also help to prevent boredom. The child can benefit by expressing his fears about hospital during lessons, either in discussion, in acting out his fears or in drawing or writing. School is an essential part of rehabilitation of the sick child.

In hospitals, lessons cannot be controlled as they would normally be, and this sometimes makes the teacher's job difficult and frustrating. Ward staff need to appreciate the importance of schooling for children in hospital, to understand the teacher's role and to give her all the support they can. Many teachers welcome nurses who will help the children with their lessons (with guidance from the teacher), for instance by listening to a child reading.

REFERENCES AND FURTHER READING

Communicating
Chapman E K 1978 Visually handicapped children and young people. Routledge, London

Nolan M, Tucker I 1981 The hearing impaired child and the family. Souvenir Press, London

McCaffery M 1979 Nursing management of the patient with pain. Lippincott, Philadelphia

Playing

Lear R 1977 Play helps: toys and activities for handicapped children. Heinemann, London

Newsom J, Newsom E 1979 Toys and playthings. Allen & Unwin, London

Weller B F 1980 Helping sick children play. Baillière Tindall, London

Eating
  Infant feeding
  Weaning
  Children and food
  Assessment and
    identification of
    problems
  Practical procedures
  Failure to thrive
  Care of the child with
    'failure to thrive'
Drinking
  Assessment and
    identification of
    problems

Practical procedures
Care of the baby with
  diarrhoea causing
  dehydration
Eliminating
  Assessment and
    identification of
    problems
  Practical procedures
  Care of the child with
    nephrotic syndrome
    causing oedema

9

Eating, drinking, eliminating

EATING

An adequate and nutritious diet is more important for children than for adults because children's reserves are smaller, and severe undernutrition in infancy has a detrimental effect on physical and intellectual development. Some children with malnutrition in the UK are obese and those whose diet consists mainly of junk foods are at risk of undernutrition.

INFANT FEEDING

The infant is wholly dependent on milk for the first 3 or 4 months of life. Breast milk is manufactured for babies and therefore suits their requirements perfectly. Cow's milk is perfect for calves but can be adapted to become a satisfactory substitute for babies. Mothers who cannot or do not wish to breast feed can therefore be reassured that artificial feeding is a satisfactory alternative.

Breast feeding

If mothers wish to breast feed, they are encouraged to do so, for the benefits are considerable:

— the constituents are suited to the baby's digestive system
— the protein content is more digestible because there is less casein which makes indigestible curds
— the milk is sterile, needs no preparation and is always available at the correct temperature
— mother and baby find it satisfying
— bonding between mother and baby is enhanced
— it is cheaper
— it contains immunoglobulins which give some protection against bowel infection
— antibacterial factors and the acid stools of the breast fed baby are thought to reduce the risk of gastro-enteritis
— it is safer for the baby in unhygienic conditions or where the mother is incapable of making feeds up correctly.

Occasionally breast feeding is contra-indicated or impossible because of the mother's physical condition or because the baby cannot suck normally.

Helping a mother who is breast feeding

Breast feeding does not come automatically to many women and new mothers need support and practical help until feeding is well established. The new baby often needs help in latching on to the nipple correctly, with his gums over the areola, and the mother also needs to learn how to help him.

The mother should be given privacy and if possible a peaceful situation in which to feed her baby. The baby's napkin should be changed and the mother relaxed and in a comfortable position. The mother starts each feed on alternate sides, for the baby tends to take more milk from the first breast when he is most hungry. It is important that the breasts are emptied regularly for stasis of milk may cause inflammation.

The baby sucks for about 10 minutes on each side, possibly for longer. He usually needs winding once or twice during the feed as well as afterwards. Nursing mothers should be offered a drink whilst feeding for they require extra fluids and are often thirsty at this time.

Artificial feeding

Many mothers bottle feed their babies because they consider it convenient and less restricting, or because they want to return to work. Some dislike the idea of breast feeding and others prefer to see the milk disappearing into the baby. Father can also be more involved by helping with feeding.

Artifical milk feeds may cause hypernatraemia and hypocalcaemia in some young babies due to differences in levels of sodium, calcium and phosphate in cow's milk. This is more likely to occur when feeds are made too strong by adding more than the recommended amount of milk powder.

Which milk?

Commercially produced modified infant milks are now recommended for all babies up to 6 months, for these milks are most like human milk. There are many brands which are very similar in content and all contain added vitamins.

Table 9.1 Comparison of human and cow's milk (g/100ml)

	Human milk	Cow's milk
Carbohydrate	7.0	4.8
Fat	3.8	3.7
Protein	1.2	3.4
Sodium (mg/100 ml)	15	50
Phosphorus (mg/100 ml)	15	99

How much milk?

As a general guide the daily requirement (for 24 hours) may be taken as 150 ml per kilogram of body weight, this amount being divided equally into the number of feeds taken. Feeds for underweight babies are usually calculated on expected weight, and energy requirements are only calculated when there is a specific problem.

Preparing a feed

The work area must be clean. All equipment used should have been sterilised by immersing in a hypochlorite solution (using tablets or Milton) for 30 minutes or failing that, boiling for 10 minutes would normally be adequate. Hands should be washed before making up feeds. The milk powder is measured in the scoop provided with the milk, for the scoops vary in size. It is filled with powder without being pressed down, and then levelled off with a knife. The instructions on the packet should be followed and extra scoops must never be added: cooled boiled water is used to make up the feed. After use, bottles are rinsed in cold water, thoroughly washed in warm water and detergent using a bottle brush, then rinsed and sterilised. Teats may be treated similarly.

Feeding the infant

Activities such as bathing are better performed before the baby is fed. He should be comfortable and have a clean napkin. The feed is heated by placing the bottle in a jug of hot water or it may be given at room temperature, but never straight from the refrigerator. The temperature of the milk is tested by allowing a drop of milk to fall onto the forearm. It should feel comfortably warm. The hole in the teat should allow a steady drop rate of one per second and it can be enlarged by using the end of a needle heated in a flame.

The baby is held comfortably in the crook of the arm while he feeds, and never left in his cot with the bottle propped up.

He needs the physical contact which feeding provides and whenever possible, a little time should be spent with him afterwards, talking and playing with him. One or two breaks are necessary for the baby to bring up his wind. An upright position, sitting on the adult's knee or over the shoulder, helps the baby to 'burp'.

Most babies take their feeds in 20 to 30 minutes. If a baby is slower than this, advice should be sought. The baby is placed back in his cot on alternate sides or prone. If he cries between feeds, he may well be thirsty and often settles after a drink of boiled water or fruit juice.

WEANING

Weaning from milk to a mixed diet is usually started at 4 to 5 months of age. There is no known advantage in starting earlier and there may be disadvantages. Weaning involves learning to feed from a spoon, to eat solid food, and to tolerate and enjoy different flavours. The process is very gradual but by the time the baby is 1 year old, he should be eating small amounts of the family meal, finely chopped.

Guidelines for weaning

1. Start with very small amounts (2 teaspoonfuls) of almost-liquid food. Broth, vegetable purée, and cereal mixed with some of the baby's milk, are all suitable. Increase the amount gradually.

2. Introduce one new food at a time and let the baby get used to it for a few days before introducing another one.

3. The food is often given before the milk feed, presuming that he takes it better when he is hungry. Some babies take it better afterwards. Consult the baby.

4. Feed the baby with a spoon, never give cereal or other solids in the baby's bottle.

5. Start with solids at one feed and gradually increase and

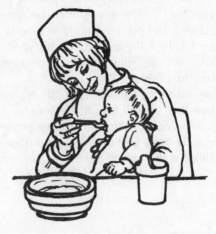

Weaning diet

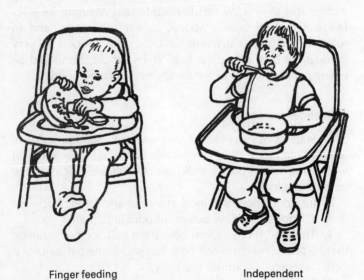

Finger feeding   Independent

Fig. 9.1 Weaning is a gradual process.

extend these to other feed times. Reduce the amount of milk accordingly and when taking sufficient solid food, offer boiled water or fruit juice instead of milk at the main meal.

6. Never add salt or sugar to the baby's food, and do not adjust it to the adult's taste. There is sufficient salt and sugar in the food content.

7. Thicken the food gradually and introduce lumps as the baby becomes accustomed to thicker food.

8. If the baby shows an obvious dislike for a food, omit it for a few weeks and then try it again.

5–12 months

The baby is now old enough to enjoy sucking, gnawing or chewing on large pieces of apple or carrot. He is less likely to choke on large pieces but should never be left alone with them. The baby learns to chew at around 5 months so lumps should be introduced into his food gradually. He starts to finger feed and enjoys small pieces of food with which he can feed himself. He learns to drink from a cup but can be independent using a teacher beaker with a spout and lid, and his mother will be less anxious about the carpet. By 10 months he is able to eat minced food and will try to use a spoon though he has to use his fingers to get the food to his mouth.

Vitamins

A child who is definitely receiving an adequate diet does not need additional vitamins. Vitamin deficiency is uncommon in the UK but may occur in recently weaned infants who no longer have fortified milk, in immigrant families, vegetarians and those whose diet is inadequate. Vitamin preparations are available at reduced prices for infants and young children and free of charge in some circumstances. Children's vitamin drops are recommended from the age of 1 month up to 2 years and preferably up to 5 years.

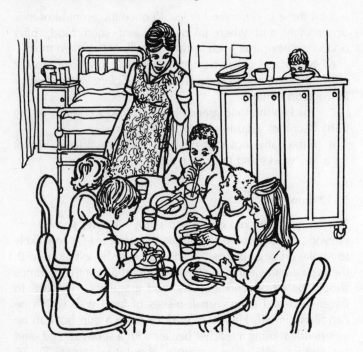

Fig. 9.2 Mealtimes—a social occasion.

CHILDREN AND FOOD

Eating habits, established in early childhood, tend to continue into adult life so 'no added sugar or salt' when weaning the baby may have far reaching effects. Attitudes and behaviour are catching and children benefit if at least one meal each day is eaten as a family meal. In hospital they eat better if they are all sitting at a table together, including toddlers and handicapped children. Interruptions during meals are less likely if the child has been to the lavatory beforehand and he should also be taught to wash his hands before eating. Cutlery and crockery should be a suitable size for the child and helpings should be appropiate for the child's appetite. No child should be forced to eat but encouragement is often necessary.

A child, who looks healthy, is active and growing normally, is eating an adequate diet although toddlers particularly tend to cause their mothers considerable anxiety with their food fads. The child often refuses food or eats one particular food for several days but shows no ill effects. When a child refuses food, the plate should be removed without fuss and the next course may be given or he may wait until the next meal. If little attention is paid and snacks between meals are avoided, the problem is usually overcome quite quickly. In hospital special allowance may be made for the sick child who may be given more of his favourite foods.

ASSESSMENT AND IDENTIFICATION OF PROBLEMS

Problems related to infant feeding cause mothers great anxiety but are not usually serious. Mother and baby may be admitted to hospital and the mother's feeding technique is observed. This assessment gives much more information than asking the mother how she feeds the baby. Problems are identified, often it is confidence that the mother needs and reassurance can be given.

Vomiting

Children are more likely to vomit and often less concerned than adults. The frequency and timing of vomiting should be noted. It may be associated with food or occur on days when school is stressful. The content of the vomitus may provide unexpected evidence of overeating or of tablets swallowed. Other observations are similar to those of adults but the volume may be assessed and measured where possible.

Possetting

Babies sometimes bring up a small amount of milk with wind which is called possetting. It is not the same as vomiting and is harmless.

Regurgitation

This is different in that the baby brings up slightly more milk either immediately after a feed or some time later. This is also harmless though messy. Regurgitation may be reduced by 'winding' the baby more thoroughly or by reducing the air swallowed. Excessive air is swallowed when feeds are taken too quickly or when crying is prolonged before a feed. No treatment is necessary but thickening the feed and sitting the baby up after feeds helps to reduce it.

Appetite

Appetite is not always a reliable guide to the child's state of health, although it is usually affected when the child is ill. A worried mother reporting that her toddler has not eaten for weeks may have overlooked that the child has taken an adequate diet between meals. If there is uncertainty about the child's health and diet, a food chart is kept so that total intake over several days is recorded. Toddlers who are reluctant to eat do not starve themselves, unlike the adolescents with anorexia nervosa who will go to any lengths to avoid eating.

Inability to feed

Sucking is hard work and sick infants tire quickly and have not the strength to take sufficient milk, so nasogastric tube feeding is often used. Infants who are tube fed include those who are breathless, due to cardiac or respiratory problems, pre-term babies who are unable to suck, and those weakened by a debilitating disease who might inhale milk. The unconscious child may be tube fed for a prolonged period and occasionally a sick handicapped child who is weak and has unco-ordinated movements may require tube feeds. Handicapped children eat in the normal way but may use special cutlery and require help with the spoon or with swallowing.

Feeding the handicapped child

Handicapped children often have difficulty controlling a spoon and co-ordinating mouth movements and swallowing. Speech therapists, who teach tongue and lip control, help children with feeding difficulties and advise staff on how to help them.

Correct positioning when eating is important. Whatever the child's age, he should sit with other children at the table. He should be sitting in a good position with the food on a table in front of him. Cutlery with angled handles and mugs with two handles may enable the child to be more independent.

Some handicapped children are hypersensitive to anything hard touching their lips or teeth, so a gentle touch is required when feeding them, and scraping the teeth with a spoon should be avoided. Using a firm unbreakable plastic spoon and placing it firmly on the tongue, helps to minimise the discomfort.

Swallowing liquids can be more difficult than swallowing dry food. The infant's feeds may be thickened and the teat hole enlarged. A child may take small amounts of liquid more easily from a teaspoon and stroking the neck in a downward direction on each side under the chin also aids swallowing. Development of the ability to chew is often delayed and the child may gag on lumpy food. If this happens, puréed foods should be given and solid foods introduced gradually.

The spastic child may be helped to swallow by pressure of the nurse's hand placed firmly on the chest to aid flexion of the trunk. If the food falls back into the child's throat, he should not be patted on the back, which encourages inhalation, but should bend forward.

PRACTICAL PROCEDURES

Measuring weight

Babies are always weighed naked as are all children whose weight must be accurate, for example those with oedema. Measures to ensure absolute accuracy are described under 'oedema'. Other children usually wear vest and pants or at least remove outdoor clothing and shoes. The small child who will not sit or stand on the scales may be weighed in his mother's arms. She is then weighed alone and her weight subtracted from the previous figure.

Centile charts are used to record children's height and weight. There are different charts for boys and girls and for different ages. The chart shows the normal growth curve and the middle line or median is the line above which and below which 50% of children's measurements lie. A series of measurements is more valuable than a single one.

Measuring length or height

The child under 2 years is measured lying on a flat surface or on a stadiometer which has an adjustable footboard. The child's napkin should be removed and the child's head is held still with the crown of the head against the board. His knees are pressed down, and both feet must be at right angles against the footboard with both heels touching it. The length is then read on the scale.

The older child is measured without shoes, standing with his back and heels in contact with a wall. He should stand up straight looking straight ahead without tipping his nose up. His heels must be on the ground. A right-angled board is then lowered until it touches his head. Gentle but firm traction is applied upwards under the mastoid process (Fig. 9.3) and the height is then read off the scale.

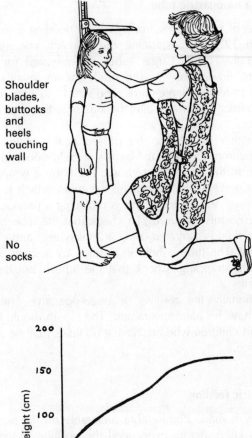

Shoulder
blades,
buttocks
and
heels
touching
wall

No
socks

Growth curve

Fig. 9.3 Measuring height.

Passing a nasogastric tube

The size of tube varies from 5FG for feeding a newborn infant to 12FG for aspirating the stomach contents of a postoperative child. Larger tubes are required for gastric washouts. Size 10FG is used orally for an infant's gastric washout to remove large curds, and size 12 to 14FG to wash out a toddler's stomach after he has ingested a poisonous substance.

The length of tube to be passed is first estimated by measuring from the tip of the baby's or child's nose to his ear and then to the tip of his sternum. The baby is wrapped up firmly to prevent him dislodging the tube, which is passed gently down one nostril. If this is replacing a previous tube, alternate nostrils are used. To check that the tube is in the stomach, fluid is aspirated using a 2 ml syringe and checked for acidity. The tube is held in position by a small piece of non-irritant strapping. Check that the tube is not distorting the nostril.

Occasionally the restless or unco-operative child may need to have his hands restrained. The mouth should be kept clean and children who are having no fluids may be allowed to suck ice.

Nasogastric feeding

The baby is made comfortable preferably on the nurse's or mother's knee. Before every feed the position of the nasogastric tube is checked by testing a small amount of aspirate for acidity. The temperature of the milk is tested, the barrel of a 10 to 20 ml syringe is attached to the tube and the milk is allowed to flow in by gravity, controlled by the height of the barrel; this should take about 10 minutes. A small amount of water is put down the tube after the milk to clear the tube. If there is any reaction such as coughing, retching or a sudden change in the baby's condition, the feed should be stopped immediately and advice sought.

The baby should be given the same attention and physical contact as the baby who is fed normally. He may benefit from being sat up for a few minutes after the feed to bring up any wind. The amount of milk and the route, whether given orally or by tube, is recorded on the feed chart.

FAILURE TO THRIVE

Young children are not infrequently admitted for investigation of this condition. The child does not appear to be growing normally or is underweight for his age or both. Accurate measurements of height and weight need to be recorded on a centile chart over a period of time in order to confirm this. The child who is perfectly healthy but small for his age may have growth hormone deficiency which can be treated by injections of the hormone. Investigations may be necessary to exclude the more unusual causes of failure to thrive such as chronic infection, congenital heart disease, renal failure or malabsorption.

In many cases the child's physical problems are found to be due to inadequate care in the home or emotional deprivation. The family's problems are often considerable and this subject is discussed in more detail in Chapter 12.

CARE OF THE CHILD WITH 'FAILURE TO THRIVE' CAUSED BY PHYSICAL AND EMOTIONAL DEPRIVATION

Problems: small and underweight, insecure, delayed development, parents with problems.

Small and underweight

Admitting the child to hospital enables his physical condition to be assessed. Height and weight are recorded on centile charts and are compared with the average for his age. If the measurements are below the 3rd centile, they are considered abnormal, although serial measurements over a period of time will be continued to provide more information. Any problems about infant feeding or diet which the parents have reported are assessed. They may say that the child will not eat what they give him, so as well as asking the parents what food they offer the child, his behaviour is assessed at meal-times.

Insecure

Relationships within the family are noted and particularly the parents' attitudes to the child. They may appear uninterested, or caring but ignorant about the child's needs. The emotionally deprived toddler tends to attract staff and visitors to him as he holds his arms out to be picked up, but being picked up constantly by strangers does not help him. The number of staff caring for the child should be strictly limited. He needs a familiar caretaker to look after him, play with him, cuddle and talk to him. In this way he can develop some security and the change in the child, within a short period of time, can be dramatic.

Delayed development

With the care described, the child's condition usually improves. He eats well, gains weight and his rate of development may accelerate remarkably and delayed milestones are achieved. Over a longer period the child's height also catches up unless the period of deprivation has been prolonged.

Parents' problems

The mother often needs as much help as the child and a trusting relationship between mother and staff is necessary if the staff are to be of any help. Parents should be encouraged to visit, to talk to staff and to be involved in the child's care. The mother may need emotional support and encouragement. Supervision and help given by staff may enable her to cope better with practical care. The parents may also need help in learning how to play with the child.

The child's admission gives the mother a break and the family a chance to sort out some of their problems. Help in hospital is provided by the social worker and in the community by professional staff and voluntary organisations who give practical help, support and advice in the home.

DRINKING

An adequate fluid intake is important for children, especially for babies and young children, because they are particularly susceptible to dehydration. The baby's daily fluid intake is 15% of total body fluid compared with the adult's which is 5%. In practical terms the baby's intake of milk based on his weight is equal to an adult drinking 10 litres of fluid a day.

The baby's kidney is immature at birth and unable to concentrate urine. It is therefore inefficient in excreting waste products of metabolism, added to which the baby's metabolic rate is higher than an adult's. He also has a larger surface area to volume ratio.

ASSESSMENT AND IDENTIFICATION OF PROBLEMS

Many sick children do not require to have their fluid intake recorded, but staff should check that all children in the ward

Table 9.2 Body water as % of weight

Body water	Adult		Child	
Extracellular	20%	} = 60%	38%	} = 76%
Intracellular	40%		38%	
Non-water	40%		24%	

are drinking enough. Particular note should be taken that cups and mugs removed at the end of meals are empty. Ideally the child's nurse should give him his food and supervise his meal so that she knows how much he has taken. When the fluid intake is recorded, the amount taken should be recorded after it has been drunk and not when it is given.

Reluctance to drink

Persuading a sick child to drink when he would rather not is reputed to be one of the most challenging tasks in children's nursing. The child's mother may be the best person to help, as parents know the child's preferences. If a parent is not resident a record of likes and dislikes is essential. The information is most useful if it is hung at the bottom of the cot, readily accessible.

The child should choose what he would like to drink bearing in mind any restrictions imposed by his condition. He may be offered a variety of flavours in a hot or cold drink—milk shakes, Marmite, different types of fruit juice or squash. Fizzy drinks such as lemonade and Coca-cola are often popular and may be offered unless the gaseous content would cause problems. Some quite young children enjoy a cup of tea.

The child may prefer to use his own mug, a special cup, a straw or even a spoon, and again he should be able to choose. A small toddler may be willing to take more from a feeding bottle. Liquid in a small glass seems less to a young child than the same amount in a large one, so he may be more inclined to take it.

Foods such as soups, jelly, ice-cream, iced lollies and custard may be used to boost the fluid intake and milk on cereals is often more acceptable than when offered on its own.

A game or a story may be used to encourage the child to drink, or he may be persuaded to finish his drink in order to see a picture at the bottom of the mug. Children may enjoy competing against each other to finish their drinks, and young children will often follow suit when they see others drinking.

An explanation about the reason for having to drink extra fluids should usually be given to children and may encourage them. They may also complete their own fluid charts, and if unable to write, they may illustrate it or stick on stars.

Children with stomatitis or tonsillitis need extra fluids but have great difficulty in drinking. A mouthwash beforehand may help and a straw may be preferred to a mug. Acid and strongly flavoured fluids should be avoided for they aggravate the soreness, and make the swollen glands of mumps more painful.

Inadequate fluid intake

The child's mouth is dry and his skin loses its natural bloom and feels dry. His eyes are sunken giving him a hollow-eyed appearance and he is lethargic. The infant's fontanelle is depressed. Urine is concentrated and the output low.

Dehydration

The higher percentage of body water in the infant and other factors already mentioned make him most vulnerable to dehydration and electrolyte imbalance. One of the commonest causes is gastro-enteritis with its classical symptoms of vomiting and watery stools.

Mild dehydration is treated by discontinuing milk and any diet and giving clear fluids for 24 hours. Boiled water can be used but proprietary preparations of an electrolyte mixture are available which are convenient and benefit the child. Milk feeds are re-introduced gradually. If there is any doubt about the child's condition, medical advice should be sought without delay.

PRACTICAL PROCEDURES

Intravenous therapy in children

The main differences from adult care relate to the sites used for intravenous (IV) infusion, the greater accuracy required in giving small amounts of IV fluid, the increased risk of overloading the child's circulating blood volume (300 ml in the newborn) and the restraint which may be required to keep the cannula in position.

Sites used for intravenous therapy

A scalp vein is often used for infants. The area is shaved beforehand and the cannula is held in place with strapping or plaster of Paris. If a limb is used for a young child, it is restrained using a splint.

The infusion

A paediatric infusion set incorporating a burette enables precise amounts of fluid to be measured and given. Used with an infusion pump or controller, the rate of flow can be regulated accurately. This may be as little as 2 ml per hour.

Leakage of fluid into the tissues (extravasation) is a real hazard of IV therapy in children. The cannula is more likely to slip out of the vein of an active toddler, the area is confined and the child may be too young to complain about the pain. Tissue damage can also be caused by fluid leaking out into the tissues from around the cannula, again caused by the activities of the child. Sites where this is particularly likely to occur are the scalp vein, the dorsum of the hand and foot and the antecubital fossa. Substances known to damage interstitial tissues include those which are strongly acid or alkaline, cytotoxic drugs and nafcillin. Permanent damage can be caused by extravasation.

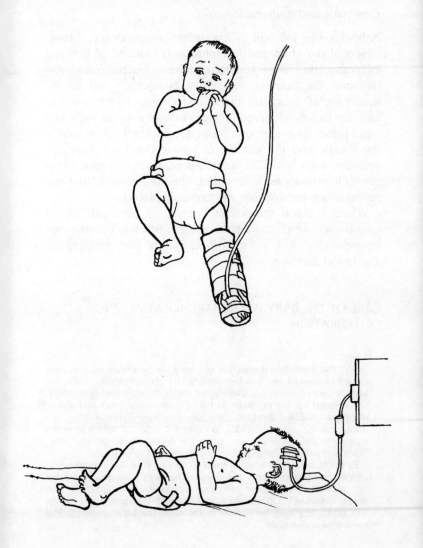

Fig. 9.4 Sites for intravenous therapy in infants.

Observing and assessing the child

Although the infusion is controlled automatically, observation of the child and the infusion is required at frequent intervals. The child's general condition, his pulse and respirations, the cannula, the site of its insertion and the infusion are all checked. Infants and young children particularly are closely observed for signs of over infusion such as a rapid pulse, dyspnoea or a moist cough. The level of fluid in the burette and the volume of intravenous fluid given are recorded each hour. The total fluid intake, and output too in some circumstances, is recorded. The nurse ensures that any restraints are comfortable and correctly placed.

When a blood transfusion is given, a paediatric blood infusion set, which has a filter, is used. Baseline observations beforehand include pulse and respiratory rate, temperature and blood pressure.

CARE OF THE BABY WITH DIARRHOEA CAUSING DEHYDRATION

Tracy
Tracy, the 3-month-old daughter of young inexperienced parents, was rushed to hospital one Sunday morning with gastro-enteritis. Tracy had been fit up to the previous evening but during the night had been fretful. She vomited her 6 a.m. bottle and shortly afterwards developed watery diarrhoea. Within a short time, the baby had passed several more fluid stools and the parents decided to contact the doctor, which involved walking to the telephone box. When the doctor arrived an hour later, Tracy was pale and drowsy.

By the time Tracy reached hospital 40 minutes later, her condition was critical. She was limp and unresponsive, her eyes were glazed and her skin mottled due to poor peripheral circulation. Her fontanelle was deeply depressed. On admission she weighed 5 kilograms which was 900 grams less than her weight in the clinic the previous week. Her parents were distraught.

Severely dehydrated babies require urgent admission to hospital, for delay may result in permanent handicap or death.

Problems: rapid pulse due to dehydration, reduced level of consciousness, infection, sore buttocks, potential damage to brain and kidneys, inexperienced and distraught parents.

Dehydration, reduced level of consciousness

An intravenous infusion is set up immediately. Normal saline is given initially followed by an electrolyte solution to correct the abnormal blood electrolyte levels. Nothing is given orally. The baby's pulse rate and volume, respirations, colour and level of consciousness are constantly observed and ½ hourly observations recorded. Temperature and blood pressure are also taken. An accurate fluid balance chart is essential and a urine bag is applied so that urine volume can be measured. Vomiting and bowel actions are charted and the volume measured or an estimate made and recorded as such.

Rehydrating the infant is synonymous with treating the baby's shocked condition. Plasma is sometimes given as the first intravenous fluid. As the baby improves, the pulse slows and becomes stronger, his colour improves and he becomes more responsive.

When the baby's condition has improved and there is no further diarrhoea or vomiting, oral feeding is re-introduced gradually. Small amounts of ½ strength milk are given initially, gradually increasing to normal amounts of full strength milk.

Infection

Gastro-enteritis is usually caused by a virus and easily spreads to other young children. The child is nursed in a cubicle and cared for by one nurse on each shift. Precautions for enteric infection are taken.

Sore buttocks

The buttocks and peri-anal area often become sore due to the frequent loose stools. The skin should be kept clean by washing and gentle thorough drying. A barrier cream helps to prevent soreness.

Complications

Renal failure and brain damage can occur as a result of severe dehydration. Continuing oliguria, twitching, fits and abnormal responses or movements are serious signs. In most cases, the baby makes a complete recovery quite quickly.

Inexperienced and distraught parents

The parents are comforted and supported. They are encouraged to stay with the baby and are instructed about barrier nursing. Once the baby's condition improves, the mother may take over his care. This provides an opportunity to discuss infant feeding and to check that she understands the importance of good hygiene and sterile feeding equipment. Gastro-enteritis is more common in underprivileged homes.

ELIMINATING

An important task for the toddler is to learn to use his pot, that is to be toilet trained. Between 18 months and 2 years the child's nervous system is usually sufficiently developed for him to learn to control sphincter muscles and to interpret sensations from a full bladder. The child may have been put on his pot much earlier and if his mother has timed this to coincide with his normal times of bowel action, she will have reduced the washing but the child is not truly trained.

Between 18 months and 2 years most children are happy to use the pot. Learning to manage it himself gives the child a greater independence which he enjoys at this age. Initially, putting the child on the pot frequently, combined with his mother's encouragement, usually gets results. The child is proud to produce something for his mother and her praise is all important. If she is relaxed and encouraging, pleased with his offering and ignores accidents he will be dry during the day quite quickly.

Any anxiety in the mother is soon picked up by the child who may see non-co-operation on his part as a method of gaining more attention. This could then become an emotionally charged situation. Most children are dry during the day by 3 years and during the night by 4 years.

ASSESSMENT AND IDENTIFICATION OF PROBLEMS

Stools

The newborn baby's stools are called meconium, a green-black sticky substance which changes to soft mustard coloured stools when breast feeding is established.

The consistency, colour and content of stools should be noted and if necessary a stool chart is recorded to check the frequency and nature of bowel actions. Black stools may be caused by iron medicine, and pale fatty stools are caused by malabsorption. Diarrhoea may vary from clear fluid stools to a semi-formed consistency.

Constipation

Constipation is the passage of hard stools at infrequent intervals. Infants' stools may become hard as a result of inadequate milk intake or too concentrated feeds. When the baby starts to drink cow's milk the stools become smaller, harder and less frequent. Older children are often constipated during a febrile illness. At any age the passing of hard stools may cause anal fissures which cause pain on defaecation. The child then postpones passing the next stool to avoid the pain which is often the beginning of troublesome constipation.

Other causes of constipation may be poor habits when children ignore the call to stool, or poor toilet training as a toddler. Occasionally it is due to a physical disorder such as Hirschsprung's disease.

In hospital, nursing staff have the responsibility for ensuring that children who are febrile or bedfast do not become constipated. The child's diet should contain adequate roughage, fresh fruit and fluids. Constipation should be treated by adjusting the diet and giving gentle laxatives.

Treatment of chronic constipation

The bowel is emptied by giving laxatives in high doses followed by an adjustment of diet to include high fibre foods and adequate fluids. A regular bowel habit is established with routine visits to the lavatory after main meals. The high fibre diet is explained to the parents who are encouraged to adopt it for the family. Occasionally enemas, suppositories and anal dilatation are necessary to clear the bowel but these are avoided if possible.

Urine

Appearance and smell

Children's urine may be an unexpected colour due to pigments in coloured sweets or other brightly coloured edible or inedible items. A sediment in the urine on standing is not abnormal but a smoky appearance is, and may be caused by pus or a small amount of blood.

The smell of ammonia in an unchanged napkin is due to the action of bacteria on urea and therefore not abnormal. It may indicate that the urine is concentrated or that the napkin has been left wet for too long.

Table 9.3 Urinary output (ml/24 hours)

Infant	250–600
Child	500–1000
Adolescent	500–1500

Volume of urine

Many young children have their fluid intake recorded but not necessarily their output. When a record of output is required, accuracy is essential. To measure an infant's urine, a paediatric urine bag is applied to collect the urine. Toddlers who are recently toilet trained require immediate attention at the cry 'wee-wee', for they have not the control to postpone micturition.

Older reliable children can be taught how to measure and record their own urine, and parents often take over this task. When urine has inadvertently been discarded and not measured, an estimated figure should be recorded and a note made on the chart. When recording fluid output, it is just as important to note and record when no urine has been passed.

Micturition

Small children pass small amounts of urine frequently, possibly hourly if they have recently acquired control. When the toddler is admitted, details should be recorded about toilet training and what name he uses for the toilet. Any established habits should be maintained in hospital. The nurse should be aware of the child's preference for pot or toilet, and whether the small boy stands or sits.

Children are likely to regress in hospital so young children, recently trained, are likely to lose daytime control and older children may wet the bed occasionally. Reluctance to go to the toilet or apparent difficulty in starting to micturate is most likely to be due to the strangeness of the environment.

Oedema

Oedema is distributed more generally in the child than in the adult. Swelling is most obvious around the eyes and face and also in the hands and genitalia. Daily weight is the most reliable measure of any change in oedema. The child should be weighed at the same time each day, on the same scales, without clothes. Ascites is assessed by measuring the child's abdominal girth with a tape measure daily. A mark with an indelible pen on the skin enables the measurement to be taken at the same level each day.

Blood pressure

Children's blood pressure is not recorded as frequently as in adult care but all children with renal disease have their blood pressure recorded, because of the association of renal problems and hypertension. It is also monitored before and after renal surgery. Other groups of children whose blood pressure is recorded regularly are those with a cardiac disorder and those who have suffered a head injury.

PRACTICAL PROCEDURES

Recording the blood pressure

- More disturbing and less pleasant procedures should be carried out after the blood pressure has been taken.
- The child needs to be relaxed and sitting quietly otherwise the measurement will be incorrect.
- Time is well spent talking to the child and gaining his confidence.
- The correct size of cuff covers approximately two-thirds of the child's upper arm. A wider cuff gives a false low reading and a narrower one gives an abnormally high figure.
- The same sized cuff should be used each time and its size recorded on the child's chart.

- The inflated inner cuff should encircle the arm and the outer cloth cover should not be creased.

The sounds of the child's blood pressure are not always easy to hear, especially in young children. The Doppler method, an alternative method of taking the blood pressure, has an amplifier incorporated in the cuff which makes the sound audible. Digital blood pressure monitors may be used for frequent recordings.

Obtaining clean specimens of urine

Obtaining uncontaminated specimens of urine from infants and toddlers is always difficult. Different methods have been devised but usually it has to be a 'clean' rather than a midstream specimen.

Before a urine specimen is obtained for culture and sensitivity regardless of the method used to obtain it, the genitalia are first washed with soap and water, rinsed and dried. Washing is repeated using clean water and the area dried with sterile wool swabs. Cleaning is from front to back, using a fresh swab each time.

Urine bag specimen (infants and toddlers)

The cleaning procedure includes the buttocks and groins and the whole area should be thoroughly dried otherwise the bag will not adhere to the skin. No powder or cream should be applied. With the child's legs separated, the perineal area is stretched and the sticky surface of the paediatric urine bag is applied to this area first, ensuring that the anus remains exposed (outside the bag) and that the skin is not puckered. The bag is pressed into position and should then be leak proof. A napkin may be applied loosely over the bag which should be checked ½ hourly so that the specimen is removed with the minimum of delay.

Thorough cleaning of the area beforehand, speedy removal and careful transfer of urine to a specimen bottle reduces the risk of contamination and inaccurate results, which can result in children being treated for a non-existent urinary tract infection.

An alternative method for infants is a suprapubic puncture of the bladder through the abdominal wall. This sterile procedure ensures that the specimen is uncontaminated. The doctor wears sterile gloves and requires equipment to clean the area, a 20 ml syringe and a needle.

A third method is to obtain a 'clean catch' specimen from a baby during or immediately after a feed. The baby is held over a clean receiver while he is fed, and longer if necessary! Most older children can manage mid-stream specimens (MSU) if instructed though some require supervision. The nurse may be able to catch an MSU from a small child, otherwise a whole 'clean specimen' is the only alternative.

Catheterisation

This method is rarely used to collect a urine sample unless the catheter is already in position for another purpose. When catheterising children, forceps are not used to hold the catheter but sterile gloves are worn instead. Spare catheters should be available, for the urethral orifice is not easy to see and the catheter may enter the vagina.

Many girls who have spina bifida and no normal bladder function have intermittent catheterisation at home. This is a clean and not a sterile procedure which the mother performs until the child is old enough to catheterise herself. The bladder is emptied at regular intervals, say 4 hourly, which helps to reduce urinary infection.

CARE OF THE CHILD WITH NEPHROTIC SYNDROME CAUSING OEDEMA

A child admitted to hospital with gross oedema is likely to have nephrotic syndrome which usually affects children bet-

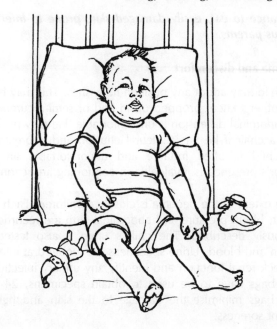

Fig. 9.5 The oedematous child.

ween 1 and 5 years of age. This syndrome occurs when large amounts of protein are lost in the urine resulting in hypo-proteinaemia which causes oedema. The reason why the glomerular membrane leaks protein is unknown. There are various forms of the disease and children recover completely from most of them. Steroid therapy is effective in many cases and is continued for some time. Relapses may occur necessitating further treatment.

The child's face is so puffy that he may be unrecognisable and hardly able to see, due to the peri-orbital swelling. The scrotum and hands are usually very swollen and ascites is common. The child is irritable, uncomfortable and anorexic.

Problems: oedema and discomfort, poor urinary output,

reluctance to eat, easily damaged skin, prone to infection, anxious parents.

Oedema and discomfort

The child may adopt any position he wishes. This may be on his mother's knee, propped up in bed or semi-recumbent if the abdominal distension is uncomfortable. He may prefer to sit in a chair if he has a pleural effusion and is breathless. The child is often irritable and uncomfortable and his mother's presence is invaluable in comforting and caring for him.

The extent of the oedema is closely monitored. Each day, weight, blood pressure and abdominal girth are recorded as previously described. The child's urine is also tested for protein and blood. Urine specimens are required at intervals to check renal function and identify any urinary infection. If urine bags have to be used to obtain specimens, 24-hour urine bags minimise the damage to the skin and help to prevent soreness.

Poor urinary output

Fluids are not normally restricted unless oliguria is marked and the blood urea rises. The fluid intake and output must be recorded accurately. After some days a diuresis occurs spontaneously or as a result of treatment with steroids and the oedema disappears.

Reluctance to eat

The child's diet should be high protein and low salt but this does not always suit the anorexic toddler who only wants crisps and cheese on toast. Apart from salty foods which should be excluded, the child may be given what he asks for, when he wants it. Set meals at routine times are often rejected, and it is a relief to see him eat anything on difficult days.

Easily damaged skin

The child's oedematous tissues break down easily, so he is best nursed on a sheepskin and his position changed at least 2 hourly. The skin must be kept clean and dry, particularly the skin folds and under the scrotum which is likely to become sore through pressure. The skin should be handled gently, and patted rather than rubbed dry. Red or sore areas should be treated at once.

Prone to infection

The child with nephrotic syndrome is susceptible to infection. 4 hourly temperature recordings and daily assessment of the child's condition identify early signs of infection. The child is particularly prone to pneumonia and peritonitis.

Anxious parents

Parents play an important part in the care of their child with nephrotic syndrome and require support and reassurance. They need a full explanation about the condition and the child's care both in hospital and afterwards. They measure and record fluid intake and output, comfort the child and persuade him to eat. After discharge they observe for any recurrence of oedema in the child and test his urine for protein.

REFERENCES AND FURTHER READING

Eating
General Nursing Council 1982 Aspects of sick children's nursing: a learning package. GNC for England and Wales (now English National Board), London, Study Unit 13
Oppe T E (Chairman) 1980 Present day practice in infant feeding 1980 DHSS No. 20 Report on health and social subjects. HMSO, London

Personal cleansing and
    dressing
  Assessment and
      identification of
      problems
  Practical procedures
  Care of the child with
      eczema causing an
      irritable skin
Mobilising
  Assessment and
      identification of
      problems
  Practical procedures

Care of the child
    confined to bed
  Combined home and
      hospital care for
      the immobilised
      child
Pre- and postoperative
  care
  Preparation for
      hospital
  Pre-operative care
  Postoperative care
  Care of the child
      undergoing
      tonsillectomy

10

Personal cleansing and dressing, mobilising, pre- and postoperative care

PERSONAL CLEANSING AND DRESSING

The child's skin is smooth, warm and elastic and is a good indicator of health. Considering how most people react to a few spots on their face, it is not so surprising that a wide-spread skin disorder or scarring is such a handicap to a child. Other children may shrink from the child and avoid touching him or he may be so sensitive about his skin that he with-draws from other children and isolates himself.

Hygiene is not of great interest to most children though some are fastidious. Similarly some children are uncon-cerned about the clothes they wear, whereas others have to

Table 10.1 Eruption of first teeth

Central incisor	6–8 mths
Lateral incisor	7–9 mths
Canine	16–18 mths
1st molar	12–14 mths
2nd molar	20–24 mths

conform to the fashion of the day for their age. Being dressed in day clothes in hospital means that children can run around normally. They feel more comfortable and 'at home' in their own clothes, as well as looking more attractive. When hospital day clothes are worn, they should be the correct size and, if possible, selected by the child.

Dental care should start in the first year of life. The importance of daily teeth cleaning, avoiding sweet snacks between meals and regular visits to the dentist should be impressed on parents and children. Dentists record seeing children under 18 months of age who already have decayed teeth caused by frequent bathing of the teeth in sweet fruit juice and syrups. These are given by a small feeding bottle which the child can hold, or through a special type of dummy which holds a small amount of liquid.

ASSESSMENT AND IDENTIFICATION OF PROBLEMS

The skin

When taking the nursing history and assessing the child's physical state, the skin is inspected for abnormalities. The colour may indicate a problem though children who appear very pale are not necessarily anaemic. Rashes are common in children, and scratches, bruises and sore areas should all be recorded. The distribution and sites of lesions may be relevant, for example the burrows of scabies are seen in specific sites such as between the fingers and on the soles of the feet. Bruises caused by an accident are common on a toddler's legs but most unusual on the face.

Identifying skin lesions

Macule	red or brown spot, not raised above the skin, e.g. measles, freckles
Papule	small raised lesion, e.g. warts
Vesicles	small collection of fluid in or under the epidermis, e.g. herpes
Pustule	similar to vesicle but contains pus
Bullae	large vesicles which may contain serous fluid or blood, e.g. severe burns
Erythema	reddened area not raised above the skin, e.g. inflammation
Wheals	transient elevations of the skin caused by oedema in dermis, e.g. an allergic reaction
Purpura	bruising, e.g. blood disorder, injury or abuse
Petechiae	pinpoint haemorrhagic areas, e.g. blood disorders

Abnormalities of the skin observed on admission should be recorded, and those found subsequently should be reported promptly.

Cradle cap (infantile seborrhoiec dermatitis)

This usually appears in the second or third month of life as a scaly area over the anterior fontanelle. A contributory factor is the mother's reluctance to wash the 'soft spot' on the baby's head which is erroneously thought to be delicate. Application of olive oil or an ointment containing 0.5% salicylic acid softens the scales and the following morning or 1 hour later respectively, the hair is washed. The treatment is repeated if necessary. Infantile seborrhoeic dermatitis may also cause napkin rash.

Ammoniacal napkin rash

Napkin rashes are common and not always indicative of

poor care. Ammoniacal napkin rash is caused by prolonged contact of the child's skin with wet napkins. Due to bacterial action, urea is converted to ammonia creating an alkaline irritant. If the rash is severe and the child is circumcised, the glans may become ulcerated leading to scarring and stenosis of the urethral meatus. Frequent napkin changes, careful washing of the skin at every change and the application of a protective cream such as zinc and castor oil or yellow soft paraffin will help to prevent this and also cure it in the early stages.

Sore buttocks heal quickly if the skin is exposed and kept clean and dry. This may not be possible because the room must be very warm to avoid chilling. Cleansing the area is less painful if oil and cotton wool are used rather than soap and water. The use of cloth napkins is preferable to disposable napkins with a plastic backing and napkin liners are also useful in keeping the area dry. The mother's method of washing and rinsing the napkins should be checked, because patent cleansing agents or soap powder in inadequately rinsed napkins are a contributory factor.

Candidal napkin rash (thrush)

This rash can be identified by its distribution. It covers all the napkin area including the flexures and perianal area, whereas ammoniacal napkin dermatitis does not, for these areas are not in contact with the wet napkin. A swab confirms that candida is the cause of the rash which is treated with nystatin ointment.

Infested head

The presence of head lice is not necessarily a sign of neglect or a poor home and they may appear in the cleanest heads! Lice are spread only by close physical contact, when they move from one head of hair to another. The occasional louse found off the hair is injured or dying and is harmless.

Outbreaks of infested heads are common in schools and one infested head may result in half the class being affected within a few days. The same can happen in children's wards. Itching and scratching of the head are obvious signs which should alert a nurse to take a closer look. The nits (eggs) appear as white specks on the hair which may look like dandruff but are difficult to remove because they are attached to the hair by a sticky substance. Lice are often seen behind the ears and at the nape of the neck, and secondary infection through scratching may cause swelling of the occipital glands.

PRACTICAL PROCEDURES

Treatment of the infested head

Various proprietary preparations are available for the treatment of head lice; these contain malathion, carbaryl or gamma benzene hexachloride. The instructions vary slightly though the principles of the procedure are the same.

An explanation is essential for the child and the parents. The treatment should be carried out in privacy for the child's sake. The lotion is rubbed into the scalp and hair, using a cotton wool swab if desired, and ensuring that the whole scalp and all the hair are thoroughly moistened. This can be achieved by parting the hair systematically and applying the lotion to each area. The hair is then allowed to dry naturally without using a hairdryer. The hair is shampooed after a stated interval, which is 2 hours if malathion is used. The hair is then combed and the dead nits can be removed by using a fine toothcomb. For severe infestation or re-infestation the treatment may be repeated after 7 days. When a child has been treated, the parents are advised to treat the rest of the family who often need treatment as well.

Topping and tailing the baby

When the baby is not bathed, he can be 'topped and tailed' instead. This involves cleaning his face as for the bath, washing his hands, skin creases and napkin area, and, if necessary, changing his clothes. His cot may be made up with clean linen as required.

Changing the napkin

The napkin area should be thoroughly washed and dried each time a wet or soiled napkin is changed, paying special attention to the skin creases. Cotton wool balls are most convenient for cleaning the area which is then washed with soap and water and gently but thoroughly dried. A protective cream may then be applied. The used cotton wool balls and soiled napkin should be placed directly into a bin or disposal bag. Any soreness should be reported and recorded.

Bathing the infant

The baby does not need a daily bath although it is traditional to do this. 'Topping and tailing' is a satisfactory alternative and is preferred if the sick baby requires minimal handling. Bathing the baby provides an opportunity to examine his skin for signs of infection such as sticky eyes, septic spots or paronychia. When he cries or yawns his mouth should be inspected for signs of thrush which, if confirmed, is treated with oral nystatin. The baby is also weighed at this time, most conveniently after his clothes have been removed and before his bath.

Preparations include ensuring that the room temperature is sufficiently warm and draught free, and having the weighing scales to hand. They should also be balanced before they are used. A plastic apron protects the nurse's or mother's clothes and a gown may be worn if the baby is small.

Cold water is placed in the baby bath first, to prevent the bath surface becoming dangerously hot. The nurse should test the temperature of the water with her elbow to ensure that it is at body temperature.

The baby is undressed on the nurse's knee, the napkin left on and the baby wrapped in a towel. Starting with the baby's face, the eyes are cleaned from the inner canthus outwards, using a fresh swab for each wipe. The rest of the face is then cleaned and dried using cotton wool; poking inside the orifices of ear and nose is not necessary. With the baby firmly wrapped up in the towel and held firmly with his head supported, the baby's hair is washed using baby soap or shampoo. It is thoroughly rinsed and gently rubbed dry using the towel.

The napkin is removed and the buttocks cleaned if necessary with cotton wool. With a soapy hand the nurse washes the baby's body all over and she should rinse her hands

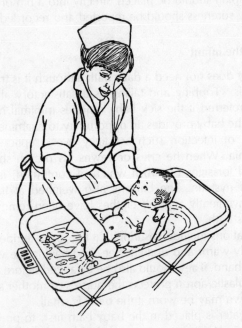

Fig. 10.1 Holding the baby safely.

before turning him over on her knee to soap his back. This provides an opportunity to inspect the skin and buttocks.

When the baby is placed in the water, the nurse should hold him firmly, at the same time supporting his head. She should continue to do this while the baby enjoys splashing or playing with his bath toys.

The baby's skin should be thoroughly dried; baby powder is used sparingly, for too much causes excessive grittiness and soreness in the skin folds. The baby should not be exposed unnecessarily nor the procedure prolonged, for he soon becomes chilled.

Bathing the child in the bathroom

When possible, the child's bath is arranged to suit the parents, so that they can bath the child at a time convenient to them. The bathroom should be warm, and staff should avoid walking in and out. A little cold water is run in first to prevent the bath surface retaining undue heat and the water temperature is tested with the nurse's elbow. Young children should never be left alone in the bathroom and older children require help or at least supervision.

Some toddlers are frightened of the big bath and need reassurance and a gradual introduction to it. Smaller baths may be used which fit inside the normal bath and are less daunting for a toddler. His nervousness may be because he has never seen a bath before or because the bathroom has previously been used as a punishment. The bathing procedure is similar to that for the baby, with the same attention to skin creases. A mild soap is best for the toddler and none should be used when washing his face.

Older children are encouraged to bath themselves, supervised if necessary. Some children are quite happy to have a bath without washing and normally co-operative children may forget to wash their necks or behind their ears. The cleanliness of these areas and the nails may require checking afterwards. Adolescents may be at a stage of neglecting basic hygiene or alternatively of being preoccupied with their appearance.

Bathing the child provides a good opportunity for the nurse to get to know the child and enables her to check the child's physical condition discreetly. Hair should be brushed and combed at least twice a day and washed weekly. Visiting mothers are encouraged to take over these aspects of care.

Children should be dressed in their own clothes whenever possible. Washing these clothes sometimes causes problems for they cannot be sent to the hospital laundry and if this happens accidently, they are usually lost. Parents are generally required to wash their child's clothes at home but resident mothers may use facilities provided for them in the ward for washing and drying clothes.

Mouth care

Most children in hospital do not require special mouth care and should continue with their usual routine if it is satisfactory. Children who have never had a toothbrush should be taught how to clean their teeth and this provides an opportunity for health education of the family. Teeth should be cleaned at least twice a day, after breakfast and at bedtime after the last drink. Young children need their teeth cleaning for them; older ones are not usually thorough enough and require supervision until around 8 years of age.

In hospital, dummies are never withheld from infants or children who are used to them at home and on occasions they serve a useful purpose, for example when a baby is unable to start oral feeding but needs the opportunity to suck. The dummy in hospital is a potential source of infection and difficult to keep in one place. It should be sterilised at least once a day and can be stored in an individual container, containing a hypochlorite solution, on the child's locker. If it falls to the ground it should be thoroughly washed under running water.

Mouth toilet

Seriously ill children usually choose to have their teeth cleaned using a toothbrush and toothpaste and to use mouth-washes. Soft yellow paraffin may be applied to the lips. Mouth toilet for a child is similar to that for adults, except when the use of forceps would be dangerous. If forceps are unsuitable, as for a baby, a disposable glove is worn and the mouth is cleaned with a dental swab wrapped round the little finger.

Application of ointment

The child with a skin disorder is very conscious of his appearance and can often feel like an outcast when other children tease him or shrink from touching him. Applying ointment can be a great booster of morale as well as of benefit to the skin, if it is applied correctly. The skin should be handled confidently without reluctance and the ointment rubbed gently in.

Gloves make an artificial barrier but are necessary if the lesions are infected or if the ointment contains active in-gredients such as cortisone, which might be absorbed through the skin. Some ointments stain the fingers which may be a reason for wearing gloves. The use of a finger stall is a good compromise. Without gloves the nurse can apply the ointment more accurately, assess skin changes better and reassure the child that she is happy to touch his skin.

THE CARE OF THE CHILD WITH ECZEMA CAUSING AN IRRITABLE SKIN

Atopic eczema is a common skin disorder in childhood in which intense itchiness is the main symptom. This is caused by a vesicular rash which at its worst is oedematous, red and weeping with crusted areas, and which may become se-condarily infected through scratching. Itchiness is a distress-

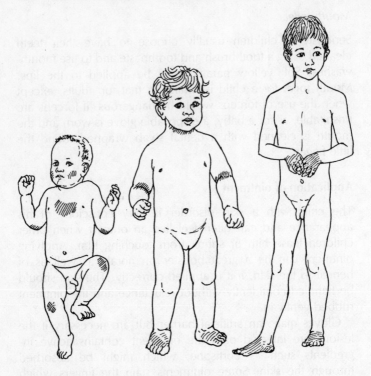

Fig. 10.2 Skin areas affected by eczema.

ing symptom which creates problems for the child as well as for his family.

Problems: intense itchiness, skin irritation, tiredness and general irritability, disfigurement, possible social isolation, tired parents.

Intense itchiness

The child may be bathed once or twice daily using an emulsifying agent. Aqueous cream may be dissolved in the water beforehand or after the child has soaked in the bath, or it may be rubbed all over the child's body before he gets into the bath. A warm bath is soothing and allows crusts to be gently removed, and the emulsifying agent helps to moisten areas of dry skin. The temperature of the bath water must not be higher than body temperature, for heat aggravates an irritable skin. Soap is best avoided but if used, it should be a simple scentless one. Bubble baths should not be used because they tend to irritate the skin further.

Having soaked in the bath, the skin is dried with a gentle dabbing action using a soft clean towel. The skin should never be rubbed or treated roughly nor should talcum powder be used. Immediately after the bath, ointments are applied as described above. If the child's scalp is affected, his hair is usually washed before the bath using a prescribed shampoo. Crusts are combed out and ointment is applied to lesions. The affected body areas are often left exposed but occlusive dressings may also be used in some circumstances.

Skin irritation

Heat, sweat or the lightest touch can irritate the skin in susceptible individuals. The room should be kept cool and the child should not be over-dressed. Clothes should be made of non-irritating materials such as cotton which is ideal. Wool should be avoided as should nylon for it induces overheating and sweating. Clothes should be light and cool without tight belt or collars which rub.

Scratching and infection is minimised by keeping the child's nails short and clean, and the child should be kept happily occupied. He is discouraged from rubbing and scratching but is never tied down. Mild sedation may be used during the day as long as it does not make the child too drowsy, and a stronger dose may be given at night. Sometimes cotton mittens or elbow splints may be worn to reduce scratching, especially at night when the child tends to scratch in his sleep. Bedclothes should be light and cotton nightwear should be worn.

Tiredness and general irritability, disfigurement and social isolation

The child should sleep more soundly with the effect of sedation and as his skin condition improves. Young children can extend their daytime rest and the older child may also like a short rest. At other times he should be encouraged to play actively but to avoid racing around so that he becomes hot and sweaty. He should be encouraged to choose an activity in which he can get absorbed, preferably using his hands. The nurse can help to restore the child's self-esteem and confidence by ensuring that she touches the child more than she normally would and avoids showing distaste in manner, speech or facial expression. The child should be encouraged to mix with other children, who will probably accept his appearance without comment if staff are setting an example. The nurse may also need to spend time playing and talking with the child, providing opportunities for him to vent his feelings of anger and frustration. From an early age the child should start to learn about his treatment and be encouraged to help. As he gets older he can manage much of the care.

Tired and despondent parents

Disturbed nights, anxiety about the child's appearance and his condition, as well as the extra attention he needs during exacerbations of eczema, all result in parents being exhausted, irritable and despondent. They too need a good night's rest. The mother is encouraged to stay with the young child to avoid the emotional trauma of separation and to learn about the treatment or any changes in it. To give the mother a break, the child's father may be able to stay for a night occasionally.

The nurse should be aware of any emotional or other problems in the child's background which might affect his condition. A confident reassuring approach is important and a close relationship between the mother and the nurse allocated to the child's care enhances this. By the time the child is discharged, one or both parents should have become competent in the child's treatment and be fully conversant with the use of ointments, skin care, night sedation and general health measures. Sensible parents are often taught to adjust the strength of the ointment according to the condition of the child's skin and to give night sedation only when necessary.

MOBILISING

The child at any age is affected by restriction of movement or total immobility. The infant depends on bodily activity to learn about himself and the world. Confined to his cot, he is deprived of normal opportunities for doing this and for normal handling and cuddling. Restraint is anathema to the toddler who is normally never still, while the immobilised schoolchild misses out socially as well, when all his friends are out in a gang or playing football.

Children confined to bed are therefore deprived of opportunities for developing, learning and enjoying themselves, and for many children immobility is one of the hardest aspects of illness to tolerate. Children's reactions to this and suggestions for helping them are discussed in Chapter 2.

Table 10.2 Types of cerebral palsy (children do not always fit neatly into one category)

Type	Movement	Damaged area of brain
Spastic	hypertonic (spastic)	cerebral motor cortex
Dyskinetic	athetosis, purposeless involuntary movements	basal ganglia
Ataxic	unco-ordinated movements and tremor	cerebellum

Many physically handicapped children have permanent problems of mobility. The child may be admitted to hospital for orthopaedic surgery involving prolonged bedrest, for a 3-week stay while his family are on holiday or because he is ill. Cerebral palsy is the commonest disabling condition in childhood and its main effects are on posture and movement. The brain damage, which causes it, is permanent and non-progressive but the disability may worsen gradually.

ASSESSMENT AND IDENTIFICATION OF PROBLEMS

Dependence of the handicapped child

The handicapped child who can move around on elbow crutches or in his wheelchair and care for himself is encouraged to maintain his independence in hospital. He is given support and help when he needs it. Some physically handicapped children have normal or above average intelligence but have difficulty speaking or expressing themselves. No physically handicapped child should be presumed to be of low intelligence because of unusual movements or speech. The child may require a longer time than usual when replying to a question or in conversation. The nursing assessment should include details of his basic problems and the help he requires as well as the effects of the disorder which necessitates hospital care.

Sitting (handicapped)

The handicapped child may spend most of his time sitting either in his wheelchair or elsewhere. He should sit in a controlled position, with both feet flat on the ground or on a box if his feet do not reach the ground. He should sit up straight, well back in the chair with the whole of his back supported. If he lacks head control, his head must be supported as well. Slipping down the chair or slouching should be avoided. An anti-slip mat on the chair may be effective and some wheelchairs have a pommel in the middle of the seat to help the child maintain an upright position and to prevent slipping. To relieve pressure the child should get up, be lifted up or move slightly every 2 hours.

Standing and lying (handicapped)

The handicapped child is not helped by being held in the standing position unless he can balance and take his weight on his feet. In fact, holding a young child like this or putting him in a baby walker may actually delay walking. Correct positioning and frequent change of position is important. Lying prone or on his side enables the child to play more easily; the supine position is not good for him and should not be maintained for long periods. The best position to prevent deformity is not necessarily the most comfortable one. One part of the body affects another when positioning a handicapped child and the position of the head is particularly important, for it affects the whole body. The child's parents can be a great help to staff by handing on tips about his daily management. Specialist staff such as speech therapists and physiotherapists give helpful advice on specific problems and if the nurse is in doubt, their advice should be sought.

The immobilised child

Assessment of the immobilised child includes how he will cope with any difficulties, for example in eating if he is lying flat, and the help he will require with washing and dressing. His state of mind should be assessed and potential problems such as depression identified. There is also the problem of maintaining his independence.

The child may be moving freely in bed but not allowed to get up, or he may be on traction or immobile in a plaster cast. Problems arising from the method of immobilisation should be identified promptly.

Traction

Traction is applied in order to exert an equal pressure in opposite directions at a given point. This might be to rest a joint or to pull apart the fractured ends of a bone. In some instances such as a fracture, a 'pull' in opposite directions must be exerted at all times.

These observations relate to a child with balanced leg traction. The principles are similar for any type of traction. The traction should be inspected regularly but additionally a quick check when passing the child's bed is always worthwhile.

Points to observe

- The leg is correctly aligned, with the toe and kneecap pointing in the same direction.
- The splints are positioned correctly and not rubbing.
- The cords are all in place, for example running over pulleys, and knots secure.
- The weights are clear of the bed and hanging free.
- The foot of the bed is elevated so that the pull of the child's body matches the pull of the traction and he is not slipping either way.
- The child's foot is warm and pink and he can wriggle his toes.
- All pressure areas are in good condition.
  Daily observation necessitating removal of outer bandages
- The extension strapping is not loose or wrinkled and has not slipped.
- The colour of the limb is normal.
- The skin of the limb is in good condition. It may become dry and require oiling.
- The weight being used is correct.
- There is no soiling around extension strapping or splints.

The outer bandages are then replaced. They are fastened with strapping rather than pins. Unexpected limited movement, altered sensation or changes in colour in the limb might be due to pressure on a nerve or an artery respectively, caused by tight or unevenly applied bandages.

Specific pressure areas which may become red or sore are the malleoli, the heels, the sacral area and the elbows. When fixed traction with a Thomas splint is used, extra care is required to avoid the groin area becoming sore. The skin under the ring should be adjusted slightly by 'walking' it out from underneath at regular intervals. Padding should not be used to relieve pressure under the ring but knowledgeable adjustment of the position of the splint or of the child can relieve it.

Gallow's traction

This is a form of skin traction used for small children to immobilise a fractured femur or to help to reduce an inguinal

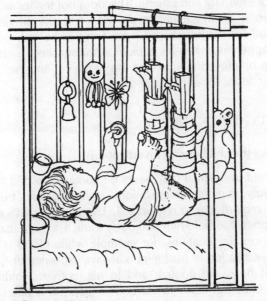

Fig. 10.3 Gallow's traction.

hernia. The child lies flat and the legs are in traction attached to a crossbar over the top of the cot.

The malleoli are protected by felt or foam padding and tincture of benzoin may be applied to the skin prior to the application of a length of extension strapping on each side of both legs. The edges of the strapping are snipped to accommodate the shape of the leg and to avoid creases. Crepe bandages are then applied to both legs from the ankle to above the knee. The legs are raised at right angles to the body and attached by extension cords to the overhead bar. Alternatively the cords may be placed over pulleys and weights attached.

The child's body provides countertraction and it is therefore essential that he lies flat and that his buttocks are clear of the mattress. A flat hand should be able to pass between the mattress and the child's buttocks. Within a week or even a few days, the child will be surprisingly mobile, leaning to the side, twisting and turning. This does not matter as long as traction is always maintained. The child should never be lifted off the mattress because traction will be lost. To avoid this happening, when his napkin or bottom sheet is changed, he can be moved towards the top of the cot and the 'pull' of the traction will be maintained.

PRACTICAL PROCEDURES

Holding the child during investigations

The child in hospital may never be confined to bed but will inevitably require investigations and possibly treatment which require him to remain still. The young child's mother often prefers to hold him, although some ask the nurse to do this in certain situations, for example while blood is taken. The investigation or treatment is always explained first, to the child if he is old enough and to his mother. Holding the child gently but firmly in the correct position is often essential for the test to be completed successfully.

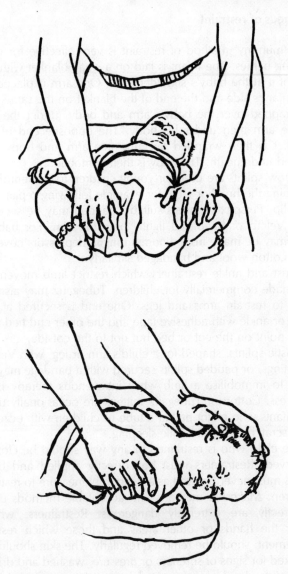

Fig. 10.4 Holding the infant for venepuncture.

Methods of restraint

The 'mummy' method of restraint is very effective for controlling babies. The infant is laid on a small blanket with the top of it at the baby's shoulder level. One arm is placed by the infant's side and the end of the blanket on the same side is wrapped over the baby's arm and body, under the opposite arm then under his body. The opposite end of the blanket is then wrapped over the free arm and body and tucked underneath. The baby is then immobile.

Elbow splints are used for young children to prevent them touching the head or face, for example following repair of a cleft lip. Perspex cylinders suitably padded may be secured with Velcro or bandaged lightly onto the arm. For babies, they may be made from wooden tongue depressors covered with cotton wool and bandaged similarly.

Wrist and ankle restrainers which restrict limb movement are made commercially for children. Tubegauz may also be used to restrain arms and legs. One end is secured at the wrist or ankle with adhesive tape and the other end tied to a fixed point on the cot or bed but not to the cotside.

Plastic splints, shaped for a child's arm or leg, with Velcro fastenings, or padded splints secured with a bandage may be used to immobilise a limb while intravenous therapy is in progress. Cotton or Tubegauz mittens are occasionally used for infants who might pull at a tube or children with eczema who scratch their skin while sleeping.

The child who is restrained in any way should be closely observed. Restrainers must be correctly applied and bandages must never be used as a temporary measure to restrain children. Makeshift methods and acceptable methods used incorrectly are extremely dangerous. Restrainers, which cover the hands or other areas and those which restrict movement, should be removed regularly. The skin should be checked for signs of soreness or pressure, washed and dried. The joints should be exercised before the restrainer is replaced.

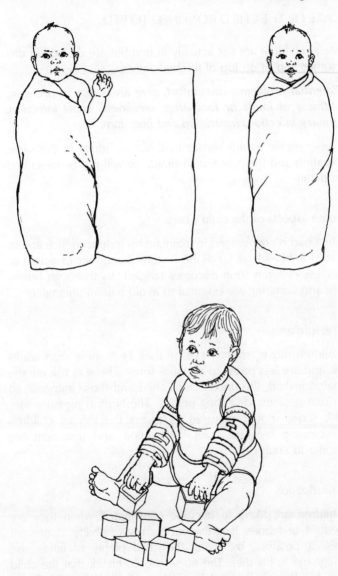

Fig. 10.5 Types of restraint.

CARE OF THE CHILD CONFINED TO BED

Many children are not actually in bed but are dressed in day clothes and sit on top of the bedclothes.

Potential problems: discomfort, sore areas due to pressure, stiffness of joints or foot drop, weakness, chest infection, urinary infection, frustration and boredom.

These problems are similar to those of adults in the same situation and the care is also similar so will not be described in detail.

Some aspects of the child's care

The child is encouraged to maintain his independence and to care for himself as far as he is able. Long hair of active or restless children soon becomes tangled, so thorough brushing and combing are essential to avoid painful untangling.

Pressure areas

Children move around in or on their beds more than adults do and are less prone to pressure sores. Those at risk are the malnourished, the unconscious child and those immobilised in one position for a long period. The Norton pressure sore risk score should be used to assess the risk of children developing pressure sores. Prevention and treatment are similar to adult care.

Constipation

Children are likely to become constipated when they are bedfast or febrile. It is the nurse's responsibility to prevent this, if possible, by giving the child plenty of fluids and roughage in his diet. The nurse should check that the child has his bowels opened regularly and aperients should be given when necessary.

Frustration and boredom

Encouraging the child to be independent, allowing him to take some decisions about his own day and enabling him to help with small jobs in the ward usually helps him. School, television, organised group activities, moving beds so that children can play together, visitors and resident parents all help to satisfy the child's needs. Staff should also be ready to listen and discuss his problems with him.

COMBINED HOME AND HOSPITAL CARE

Congenital dislocation of the hip

When this condition is diagnosed in late infancy or early childhood, the treatment may continue for a year or more. It involves an initial period of traction in hospital (Karen's position at the beginning of Chapter 1), surgery and several months' immobilisation in a hip spica during which the child is at home. This is a good example of combined home and hospital care, with parents and staff working closely together.

The parents take much of the responsibility for the child's care and for ensuring that the child's development is delayed as little as possible. A resident mother, as part of the ward team, participates in the care of the child immobilised in traction and in a plaster hip spica, and is able to continue it at home. She also gets to know the ward staff well and feels able to contact them at any time.

The parents require mobility aids such as a buggy or pushchair. A special chair is required for the child, which the father may be able to make. The child needs to be given maximum independence: he benefits from outings and mixing with other children. It is easy for hospital staff to give advice about the child's care at home, but much more difficult for the mother to follow it, when her day is already a busy one. Community and hospital staff support the family but in spite of this, parents do find the situation stressful.

Spina bifida

This is another condition which requires combined home and hospital care but in this instance it may be a heavy burden on the parents for life.

Types of spina bifida

Spina bifida occulta—an abnormality of a vertebra in which the spinous process is divided (bifid): this is often undiagnosed.

Mengingocele—the meninges herniate through the gap in the vertebra and form a sac over the spine filled with cerebrospinal fluid which may be covered with skin.

Myelomeningocele—the most serious defect in which the nerves of the spinal cord are exposed on the child's back.

The baby with a myelomeningocele requires surgery in the first 24 hours of life to close the defect and prevent further damage to the nerves. The child may have paralysis and anaesthesia of the lower limbs, hydrocephalus, and dislocated hips as well as paralysis of the bowel and bladder sphincter. He is prone to urinary infections which eventually cause renal failure and is also susceptible to pressure sores in the affected limbs.

Treatment may continue intermittently for years and involve numerous operations. The effect on the child's life and the problems for the family can be imagined.

PRE-AND POSTOPERATIVE CARE

PREPARATION FOR HOSPITAL

A child who learns about doctors and hospitals as opportunities arise at home is better prepared for a hospital stay should the occasion arise. Pre-school children may become interested when they have been taken to see the doctor, and books about hospitals often interest them. Children in nursery schools can be shown slides about going to hospital. This preparation is particularly valuable because most children are admitted as emergencies and there is no time to prepare the child.

Preparation prior to a planned admission

Children require information and emotional preparation prior to surgery. Although not always ideal, this often starts in the outpatient department when an operation is found to be necessary. The older child hears what the doctor is saying and nursing staff can expand or clarify the surgeon's explanations. The young child may overhear the adult conversation and interpret it in his own way, so an explanation is required to avoid him becoming anxious and disturbed. Otherwise young children may be told 2 weeks or so before their admission. This allows time for explanation and discussion. Stories about going into hospital are available for every age group and comics and painting books on this subject are available.

The family may be shown the ward and meet the staff prior to admission. They may be invited to visit the ward with other families in a similar situation and they may be shown a video of a child's stay in the ward. Parents and children's queries are answered and the possibility of parents staying is discussed. An information booklet about ward facilities should be sent to the parents before the child's admission.

PRE-OPERATIVE CARE

The child should be admitted to the ward by the nurse who will look after him for the rest of the day. The child does not need to be bathed immediately unless he is obviously dirty, nor does he need to change into night clothes. Certain aspects of the admission procedure (see Ch. 3) are particularly relevant before surgery:

- the child's nameband must be in place
- his weight is required for calculation of doses of pre-medication, anaesthetic and other drugs
- urine is tested to exclude diabetes
- temperature is taken to exclude infection
- any loose teeth or dental plates are recorded.

Jewellery is best removed and taken home unless the child feels strongly about it or takes responsibility for it. Nails should be checked for nail varnish which may be overlooked.

Consent for operation

The doctor talks with the parents, explains the operation and asks them to sign the consent form. A parent must sign the consent form for children under 16 years of age. If the parents are divorced, it is wise to check who has the custody of the child for that person should give consent. If the child is fostered it is usually a social worker who gives consent. Before the parents go, the nurse should check that the consent form is signed and that a telephone number or other means of contacting them is recorded in the nursing notes.

Bowel preparation is not usually required unless the operation involves the intestinal tract. If the child is thought to be constipated, glycerine suppositories may be given on the day prior to surgery.

Explanations

An explanation about the operation, suitable for the child's age, and information about what will happen afterwards, reduce apprehension and imagined horrors. Play can be used to explain to a young child about an operation (see Ch. 8). The information should be truthful with no false promises. Explaining an anaesthetic to a child is tricky. Having a 'sleep' may mean 'during the night' to a young child and make him reluctant to go to sleep at night. 'Putting to sleep' is worse because a much loved pet may have been put to sleep and never been seen again. One way of describing an anaesthetic is to say that a doctor will give 'a special sleep' so that the child will not know anything about the operation and will wake up in the ward.

Parents are encouraged to be resident with young children and if not resident, to visit on the day of operation, both before it and afterwards. This makes the child more relaxed as well as reassuring the parents.

Immediate pre-operative care

Pre-operative fasting reduces the risk of vomiting and inhalation after anaesthetic but increases the risk of hypoglycaemia, especially in young children; 6 hours without food and the last drink 4 hours before elective surgery is the usual procedure for children. Because of the risk of the infant developing dehydration and hypoglycaemia, his last milk feed is given 4 hours pre-operatively and if the operation is delayed, an intravenous infusion may be set up.

A thirsty and hungry child is likely to help himself to any fluid or food which is within reach so all food, sweets and drinks should be removed out of reach and sight of the child. A notice 'Nothing by mouth' alerts visitors and reminds staff to be watchful, as other children may also offer the child food.

The child has the usual bath on operation day. Cleanliness of nails, feet, neck and behind ears, umbilicus, and skin creases is checked, as well as the operation site. Hair should be clean. He is dressed in a cotton operation gown and if he insists on wearing his pants, as long as they are clean, they can be removed in the anaesthetic room. Distressing procedures such as shaving the hair or passing a nasogastric tube may also be carried out under anaesthetic. The child is encouraged to pass urine before he is given his premedication.

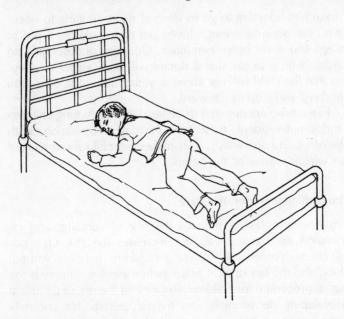

Fig. 10.6 Semi-prone position.

The child's premedication is given orally whenever possible. Young children are often given trimeprazine or diazepam for sedation and atropine to dry up the secretions, all orally.

When the child's premedication has been given, he is settled into his cot or bed where he plays quietly until he drops off to sleep. He should be observed during this time and the cotsides should be raised unless his parents are with him. A familiar nurse and the mother of the young child, if she is present, should accompany the child and his favourite toy to the theatre. If the mother is not allowed to remain while the child is anaesthetised, the nurse should stay with him. Babies need to be warmly wrapped when transferred to and from theatre and an incubator may be used for the smallest ones

POSTOPERATIVE CARE

While the child is conscious but not fully awake, constant observation is required. The airway may become obstructed by secretions and occasionally laryngospasm may occur as a result of intubation, inhalation or the effects of the anaesthetic. The child is therefore placed on the trolley in the semi-prone position with a pillow behind his back to maintain a clear airway. Oxygen and suction should be available. The nurse keeps one hand lightly on his body to reassure him and to detect any sudden movement. Some children are wide awake when they reach the ward, others sleep for hours. Analgesia is given when necessary (see p. 189).

Fluids and food

Unless contra-indicated, small amounts of water are given to the child as soon as he is fully awake. These are usually gratefully received and the child can quickly progress to a light diet within, say, 8 hours of recovery. Children seem to feel better once they have had some food. If the child vomits, he may continue to have sips of water and increase the amount more gradually. Babies usually tolerate a clear feed as soon as they are really awake and have their usual milk at the following feed.

Care of the wound

Children's wounds often require little attention apart from checking that they are not infected. Sutures are absorbable and the dressing may be a plastic spray, a waterproof plaster or the traditional gauze dressing. The child is discouraged from fiddling with the dressing and in some areas, may be given a daily bath after the operation. The area should be carefully dried with a clean towel and the wound may be covered with a plaster to protect it from rubbing.

On discharge

The child is frequently discharged within a few days, and the parents are given verbal and written instructions about after care. Details about care of the wound, bathing, exercise, sport, returning to school and any medication are included. If the parents are worried about the child, they are advised to contact their own doctor who will be sent a letter about the child's condition. The health visitor is informed if the child is under 5 years.

CARE OF THE CHILD UNDERGOING TONSILLECTOMY

This section relates specifically to tonsillectomy and should be read in conjunction with the general pre- and post-operative care already described.

Pre-operative care

Problems: anxiety of the child and mother
Potential problems: infection delaying operation or causing complications, accidental eating and drinking, postoperative complications—asphyxia, bleeding and infection.

Anxiety of child and mother

The child's anxiety is reduced if he has been adequately prepared and if his mother is able to stay with him. A friendly welcome and one nurse to whom he can relate also help him to settle into the ward. Most children admitted in a group for operation the following day soon make friends. The nurse should ask the child what he thinks is going to happen and correct any misconceptions. She may warn him that he will not be allowed breakfast the following morning.

Potential postoperative infection

During the initial nursing assessment on admission, any signs of infection are noted. A cough, a rash or a raised temperature are reported at once. The mother is asked about any contact with an infectious disease or recent immunisations.

The child has a bath on the evening prior to the operation and the child's hair should be washed unless it is known to be clean. On the morning of the operation the child has another bath when cleanliness of the neck, ears and nails is checked. The child is then dressed in a clean operation gown. The teeth should be cleaned.

Potential bleeding postoperatively

On admission the parents are asked if the child or any other family member has a bleeding tendency. If so, tests for bleeding and clotting time will be carried out. The child's haemoglobin is estimated routinely in many centres.

Postoperative care

Potential problems: asphyxia, bleeding.
Problems: sore throat and reluctance to eat and drink.

Asphyxia

The child is nursed in the semi-prone position without a pillow until he is fully conscious. In this position any blood will drain out of his mouth and his tongue cannot fall back and obstruct his airway. Suction and oxygen should be available. Colour and respirations are observed and the child should not be left unattended until he is fully conscious. He may then lie in any comfortable position. A nurse should remain in the area and his mother may be with him.

Table 10.3 The child's pulse

Age	Pulse rate/minute	Sites at which pulse may be taken
Birth	110–150	anterior fontanelle (infant)
0–1 year	100–140	temple — temporal artery (sleeping toddler)
1–5 years	80–120	*chest — apex beat (infant and toddler)
5–15 years	70–110	*wrist — radial artery
		foot — dorsal pedis artery

*most used

Bleeding

During the first 24 hours close observation is maintained for bleeding and the pulse rate is recorded ½ hourly initially. There is normally a little oozing at first and the child may vomit altered blood but this is not serious. The child's mouth can be cleaned with gauze swabs and iced water.

Signs of bleeding:

— rising pulse rate
— swallowing visible in the neck while asleep
— vomiting fresh blood
— restlessness
— pallor and occasionally abdominal pain
— fall in blood pressure (late sign).

Sore throat and reluctance to eat and drink

The sooner the child starts to swallow, the less discomfort he will have, and small amounts of iced water are given as soon as he is fully awake. These are continued at frequent intervals and the amount gradually increased. After a morning operation, most children are ready for jelly and ice cream or a light meal for tea or supper. A good fluid intake is maintained and a normal diet encouraged from the first postoperative day. Chewing and swallowing movements help to shorten the initial period of discomfort; some children take fluids and food with little complaint while others need a lot of encouragement. Paracetamol may be given for a painful throat, for earache and before meals.

If the child's condition is satisfactory on the day after the operation, he can be bathed, dressed and play quietly at the table. He is usually discharged home on the second post-operative day.

Advice to parents

Children should remain indoors for 1 week after the operation. The child should have a normal diet and plenty of fluids. If there is any bleeding from the throat, the family doctor should be called or the child may be taken back to the hospital. At this stage bleeding is rarely severe.

The family doctor may see the child before he returns to school which is usually after 2 weeks.

REFERENCES AND FURTHER READING

Mobilising
Finnie N R 1974 Handling the young cerebral palsied child at home. Heinemann, London
Harrison S P 1977 Families in stress. Royal College of Nursing, London
Roaf R, Hodkinson L J 1980 Textbook of orthopaedic nursing. Blackwell, Oxford

Pre- and postoperative care
Adamson E F S, Hull D 1984 Nursing sick children. Churchill Livingstone, Edinburgh, chs 4, 8, 9, 10, 15, 16
Balbernie R 1985 Fear is the key. Senior Nurse 3 (4): 20–22
National Association for the Welfare of Children in Hospital (NAWCH) 1980 Preparing children for hospital. Research Project, NAWCH, London

Children's ideas about
    death
Explaining to the child
    about his illness
Parents' reactions and
    feelings
Sibling reactions

11

Dying

Aspects of care of the dying which specifically relate to
children are considered in this section. The short statement
at the end of Chapter 2 entitled 'Reactions to a child's death'
is a good starting point and makes a useful introduction here.

CHILDREN'S IDEAS ABOUT DEATH

Each child has his own understanding of death which may
vary considerably from that of another child of the same age.
Therefore, it is often necessary when a child talks about
death to find out what he means. Fochtman & Folet (1982)
use Nagy's theory on the child's thoughts about death which
is helpful as a broad framework.

3–5 years

The child understands death as sleep, and thinks it is temporary. Separation, loneliness, restraint and immobility are associated with sleep and death. The child may talk about
funerals and burials in a detached way.

5–9 years

The younger child in this age group realises that death means an end to life (bodily functions) but sees it as a reversible process. 'Shall we invite Granny (who died last month) to my birthday party?' The older child accepts death more concretely but does not apply it to himself.

9–10 years

At this age death becomes personal and inevitable. The child usually accepts his parents' ideas about death and may have concepts of an after-life.

EXPLAINING TO THE CHILD ABOUT HIS ILLNESS

It is essential that the child's illness and treatment are explained to him in the same way by both parents and staff, who therefore need to agree on the approach to be taken. Every child needs to know about his illness and this includes life-threatening disease. Honesty is essential but information should not be overwhelming and can be given gradually in small pieces. Any information given to the child by parents or staff must be consistent and it is helpful to record it. Often a child's imagination can make his illness terrifying and worse than the truth.

If there is honesty, the child nearly always comes to terms with his condition more quickly and better than an adult. Honesty also maintains his security and trust in his family and in others who are looking after him. A child soon realises if he is being told lies, and will stop asking questions or ask someone else and probably receive inaccurate answers.

It is unusual for a child to ask openly 'Am I going to die?' which in any case may not mean what the adult initially understands it to mean. Asking a question in return is often the best response, for example 'What makes you ask the question?' or 'What do you mean by that question?'. There is no correct answer or one single answer, and each time a different response is required depending on the circumstances and what the child meant.

PARENTS' REACTIONS AND FEELINGS

The first shock for the parents comes when they are told about their child's illness. It is helpful if a nurse who is involved in the child's care is present so that she knows what has been said and can explain and reinforce the information later, and possibly record what has been said. The parents are told carefully and gently but as soon as they hear words like 'leukaemia' or 'cancer', they are unlikely to absorb any further information. Shock overwhelms them and they need time to digest the news. It is more satisfactory when both parents are given the information together for if it is handed on from one to the other, misunderstandings or feelings of being excluded or not being told the truth, may cause problems between the parents. The initial talk is followed up in discussions later so that the parents have an opportunity to ask questions. Information may need to be repeated several times before it is absorbed.

The first feelings of the parents are often inadequacy in that they have failed as parents and lost control of the situation, for they cannot meet the child's needs and everything is chaotic. They cannot think, and feel panic-stricken and confused. Anger, denial, fear, resentment and guilt are all normal reactions which parents will feel at some time.

As soon as possible the parents need help to resume their parental role, and to do this a partnership needs to be established between parents and staff. The parents need to pick up their role in a different way so that they can love and support the child and look after him although he is going to die. They also need to maintain normal discipline for the sick child and as normal a life as possible for the rest of the family.

Amanda

Amanda was a 13-year-old girl who was admitted to hospital with a short history of bone pain, anorexia, weight loss, swelling of her right shin and anaemia. She was found to have a rare type of tumour which might respond to treatment. Her parents agreed that a trial of chemotherapy seemed to be justified.

Amanda had one younger brother and came from a closely-knit family who had strong Christian beliefs. When the parents were told the diagnosis, they told Amanda themselves, for they felt that honesty and openness were the best approach, particularly for an intelligent girl of her age. Although obviously shattered by the diagnosis, Amanda's family seemed to cope very well.

Despite several courses of chemotherapy, tumour cells persisted in the bone marrow. The deposits of tumour cells in various bones also caused severe bone pain from about 2 months after diagnosis. An expert on pain was consulted and his advice was followed. Amanda visited the hospital on a day basis for her treatment but was admitted on two occasions in order to adjust the dose of analgesic. Her parents found episodes of severe pain extremely upsetting and hard to cope with.

After 4 months of chemotherapy and radiotherapy there was no improvement and it was decided that active treatment would be discontinued. Amanda's parents had already thought that this was inevitable and they agreed with the decision.

On her last admission to the ward, Amanda was initially nursed in the main ward which she preferred, for she enjoyed the contact with other children, especially the younger ones. Were it not for the problem of pain control, Amanda would have been nursed at home by her parents, but they felt she was better off in hospital where pain control was more easily managed and Amanda more settled as a result. On one occasion Amanda's mother shouted at a nurse angrily but later apologised. Her father was always outwardly cheerful and calm.

As Amanda's condition was deteriorating, she was moved into a single room in order to give the family some privacy and to avoid distressing the other children in the ward. Her parents continued to carry out all her care and rarely accepted offers of help. They wanted to feel that they were looking after Amanda. Good pain control was achieved by an intravenous morphine infusion which was speeded up or slowed down as Amanda requested. Her mother was apprehensive initially when doing this but with practice soon gained confidence. With the pain well-controlled and the honest and open relationship between staff and family, the staff found it very easy to enter the room and spend time chatting.

One evening Amanda asked what the lumps were on her head. While the nurse paused to think what to say, her mother calmly told her that it was her cancer. She also told her that she was not going to have any more treatment for it. Amanda indicated that she knew this meant that she was going to die and was reassured by her mother that she and her father would remain with her and that she would not be alone. The doctor was told what had been said so he went in to see Amanda to find out if she had any queries. All she wanted to ask was when would she die. He answered truthfully that he did not know but thought it would not be very long and reiterated what her mother had said about not being left alone and her parents and the nurses keeping her company. From that time she did not ask any further questions of the staff about death but was able to talk to her parents.

The following morning, the atmosphere in Amanda's room was remarkable — peaceful and happy. Amanda had told her mother that she was ready to go to Heaven to be with Jesus and she appeared much calmer. Her parents felt a great sense of relief that Amanda knew what was happening and had coped with that knowledge. They had always been honest with her but had not found a way of telling her that she was dying.

Amanda's brother was a frequent visitor. His birthday was approaching and Amanda's was 3 weeks later, so the parents thought that a joint celebration would be appropriate. This gave the family something to plan and prepare for. On the day, Amanda's bed and room were hung with decorations and balloons. Many family members and friends came to share a marvellous spread. Amanda's parents bought her a gold ring which she had wanted for a long time and the staff bought her a bracelet which enabled them to express their feelings. After the family and friends left the room many were in tears and Amanda's parents did much of the comforting.

Amanda died peacefully 1 week later with both her parents present. Looking back, Amanda's mother was pleased that her 'birthday' had been such a success and remembered with pleasure how much it had meant to Amanda.

This is not the end of the care of the family for it continued over the subsequent weeks, and contact is sometimes maintained for years.

Although the account of Amanda's last illness has been shortened and much of the detail omitted, it illustrates the approach and the type of care which a dying child and the family need. Experienced staff found caring for Amanda rewarding though distressing at times. They also felt that they had learnt much from her and her family. No two familes are alike and the approach adopted here was right for them but would not necessarily be right for another family.

Aspects of care to think about

- The parents adapted to a new role and gained great comfort in looking after Amanda.
- The parents participated in discussions and decisions about Amanda's treatment.
- The parents coped with this situation in their own way as they would any other crisis, and the staff supported them in this.
- Pain control was extremely difficult to maintain. The aim was to prevent the pain recurring, which was achieved in the final stages of the illness.
- Amanda's mother's anger which erupted against a nurse was beneficial for the mother in relieving tension. Both child and parents may feel anger which needs to come out. The nurse helped the mother by accepting the outburst and not turning away or being upset.
- Co-ordinated care was achieved by nurses, doctors and parents working closely together.
- The party provided a happy distraction and later a happy memory for the parents. Special treats and outings are often organised for children who may be close to death.

SIBLING REACTIONS

Siblings should be allowed to be sad and to grieve if they wish. Their reactions may be unpredictable.

A man whose wife had just died was trying to tell his 6-year-old son gently. The boy took it all in and looking very serious said, 'Well, Daddy, I might as well tell you. Mummy owed me 10 pence.'

When a child is seriously ill or dying, the siblings sense that something is wrong. If they are not told, family communications break down, they loose faith in their parents and become insecure, which may have far reaching effects. The siblings can be told, as the sick child is told, in small manageable bits. If they are not involved with the sick child, they may have erroneous fears about the dying child or death.

Excluding the other children from the situation and sending them away for the funeral does not help them, for it can easily be seen as rejection of them by their parents. They are also deprived of opportunities to grieve. They may think that children are disposable and they will be the next to go, or they may blame themselves for the child's death.

The child needs opportunities to express his thoughts and feelings. He may have the same feelings as adults such as anger and grief. If the sibling shares in the care of the sick child, and members of the family talk about their feelings, the child is emotionally secure and family life may be enriched.

REFERENCES AND FURTHER READING

Adamson E F S, Hull D 1984 Nursing sick children. Churchill Livingstone, Edinburgh, ch 12

Hagan A J, Buschman G P 1983 A child dies. A portrait of family grief. Aspen, USA

Kübler-Ross E 1983 On children and death. Macmillan, London

Parkes C M 1986 Bereavement. Pelican, Harmondsworth

Robbins J (ed) 1983 Caring for the dying patient and the family. Lippincott Nursing Series. Harper and Row, London

PART FOUR

A wider view

Child abuse
Hospital care of child
    with non-accidental
    injury
Social factors affecting
    hospital admission
Disadvantaged parents
Preparation for
    parenthood

12

Social problems

CHILD ABUSE

Child abuse is not a new problem but ideas on treatment of children, child rearing and punishment have changed and there is now a greater awareness of the problem. Only in the last 30 years has child abuse been fully recognised and investigated. Abused children used to be called battered babies but this term is not used today. Child abuse is the preferred name because there are several categories of abuse. Physical abuse is often called non-accidental injury (NAI) and this is the diagnosis of many of the abused children admitted to hospital.

Types of child abuse

Physical violence includes:
- bruising caused by hitting or pressure of the finger tips on the chest when the child is held and shaken, black eyes
- burns caused by cigarettes or a hot object, scalds
- scratches, bites, damaged frenulum (baby's mouth) or bruised ears (due to being boxed)

- fractures
- poisoning
- drowning and suffocating.

The most serious injuries, caused by banging the child's head or shaking him, are likely to result in subdural haematoma, permanent brain damage or death.

Physical and emotional neglect develops gradually and may pass unnoticed for many months. Physical neglect implies malnutrition, low weight for age and lack of care. Emotional neglect usually occurs with physical neglect.

Emotional abuse is a more subtle form of abuse. The child is constantly scolded, punished or ridiculed. For example, he may be made the family scapegoat and called 'Stupid' instead of his proper name. Brothers and sisters may be encouraged to tease him and he may be deprived of special treats that the others have. The scars of this type of abuse are not physical but psychological and more damaging.

Sexual abuse involves dependent children and adolescents in actions which they do not fully understand such as incest, molestation and rape, without their informed consent.

Incest is often hidden for years because the family is reluctant to report it and may in fact support it, in order to avoid disruption of family life. Reporting it affects every member of the family, causing disturbed relationships and adverse publicity. It is likely to result in legal action, unemployment, loss of family income and possibly the break-up of the family. Children of every age group, from babies to adolescents, have been involved in cases of sexual abuse.

The background to child abuse

Child abuse occurs in families from all walks of life but more so in the underprivileged. There are certain factors which the families tend to have in common:

1. The parents often have a background of emotional or physical deprivation and sometimes abuse as well.

2. The child is usually seen as 'difficult', unlovable or a disappointment.
3. There is a crisis, the 'final straw', which causes self-control to snap and rage to erupt.
4. The parents have no lifeline, that is no friends or relatives to whom they can turn when needing support, relief or advice.

The parents

The parents often seem immature, and have frequently lacked parental love themselves and had problems at every stage of life. They tend to have a poor self-image and have not learnt to form trusting relationships. They may be isolated and feel that they should cope alone, but have no inner resources to call on when a crisis occurs. If the baby is good the mother may cope, but if he cries a lot she thinks that he is showing his rejection of her as a mother. The parents may also have totally unrealistic expectations of the baby. For example they think he is being wilful at 3 months when he dirties his nappy, so they smack him. The parents' perception of the relationship between them and the child often seems to be distorted.

The child

The baby may be difficult in that he cries a lot, or does not respond readily to attention. His birth may have been difficult, he may have been premature or have a congenital defect. The baby may not match up to his mother's or father's expectations so that he is a disappointment and they take a dislike to him. Difficulties may only arise as the child grows and demands more attention and becomes a nuisance.

Developmental delay and failure to thrive is a sign of abuse in the young child. The baby or young child may be hypervigilant and abnormally co-operative for his age. The older child may have learning problems and a low capacity for enjoyment. Sexually assaulted children may have medical and sexual problems.

The crisis

When stress in the family becomes excessive the slightest mishap assumes huge proportions, violence erupts and the baby is hurt. The last straw often seems trivial to an outsider, for example the baby crying or an argument, but it precipitates a crisis and anger is vented on the child.

HOSPITAL CARE OF THE CHILD WITH NON-ACCIDENTAL INJURY

When the child has been physically abused the parents may delay bringing the child for medical attention. Their story is often unrealistic and does not match the injuries. No specific behaviour is indicative of abusing parents. They may be anxious or aggressive but may equally be quiet, casual or evasive. Often they are relieved when admission is advised.

The child is examined and a detailed history is taken by the doctor. The type and extent of the injuries are recorded, they are photographed and a full skeletal survey is carried out. Blood is examined to exclude a bleeding disorder. If NAI is suspected the child is admitted for his own safety as well as for treatment.

A Place of Safety Order is obtained if the parents will not agree to the child's admission. This is a legal document which orders that the child be detained in a place of safety for a stated number of days up to 28. The definition of a place of safety is one controlled by the local authority, a hospital or a police station. The Order is obtained by the local authority, the NSPCC or any individual who may apply to a magistrate. The applicant must produce evidence that the child is at risk.

Nursing problems: nurses' feelings, parents with problems, injuries of the child, possible emotional abuse.

Nurses' feelings

The child and his family should be welcomed to the ward in the usual way. Any indignant feelings which the nurse may have should not be apparent nor should they be allowed to affect the care of the family. This is sometimes difficult, and it may help to remind oneself that it is the parents who need the help if the child is to have a normal family life. Many staff also reflect on how frustrating children can be, and that most people have felt like hitting out, at one time or another. Staff and parents of other children in the ward should not discuss or comment on the child's condition or situation. Besides being unethical, this creates a hostile atmosphere which can be very obvious and does not help the family.

Parents with problems

The parents may be fearful or resentful in the ward. They are encouraged to visit and participate in his care but are often reluctant to do this and may visit infrequently. Staff should chat normally with them and observations are made on how often they visit and the interaction between parents and child. They are kept up to date about the child's condition. The doctor has several discussions with the parents in order to understand their problems and feelings, and to ascertain facts if possible. While the child is the subject of a Place of Safety Order, his parents cannot remove him from the hospital.

Physical injuries and possible emotional abuse

The child's general condition is assessed and injuries noted. Treatment may involve dressing skin wounds but traction might be required for a fracture, or surgery to relieve raised intracranial pressure. The child's weight and length or height are recorded and will show whether he is growing normally. If his development is delayed and his weight is below normal, physical and emotional neglect are the probable cause. The care of the child is similar to that for the child with failure to thrive (see Ch. 9).

During the child's stay in hospital, reports are compiled about the family by staff who have had contact with the family. These may include the health visitor, social worker, an officer of the NSPCC, nursery teacher, paediatrician and ward sister. The police may also be involved.

Case conference

When the investigations are complete, a case conference is held at which representatives of all the relevant services meet to discuss the family's problems. A decision is made about the child returning home or being taken into the care of the local authority. A key worker is appointed from the group, who will work closely with the family and build up a relationship with them. The child's name may also be placed on the 'at risk' register. This is a confidential register of children who have either been abused or who are in a situation where abuse is suspected.

SOCIAL FACTORS AFFECTING HOSPITAL ADMISSION

Children whose admission to hospital is related to social factors are not necessarily abused, neglected or malnourished.

Jennifer

Jennifer, aged 13 years, suffered from asthma and because of problems at home, went to a residential school for children with health problems. She went home for the holidays. Her asthma was well-controlled and caused no problem at school, but every holiday without fail, she had a severe asthmatic attack which necessitated a few days in hospital.

Jennifer's asthmatic attack may have been due to a variety of causes, but a major factor was considered to be the discord in the family which had been the reason for her going away to school in the first place.

Hayley

Hayley was 3 years old and had cystic fibrosis. Her mother had been taught how to give Hayley her daily chest exercises but Hayley's condition deteriorated rapidly because her mother carried out the physiotherapy when she felt like it and not daily as instructed. Although she appeared to understand how important it was, she was unable to keep it up.

Most parents manage to care for their children at home extremely well, and faithfully maintain any treatment ordered. Some parents are unable to cope with the added burden and the child may suffer.

Carl

Carl, aged 10 weeks, was brought to the paediatric casualty department by his unmarried mother one Saturday evening. She said that he had diarrhoea and had not taken his last feed. The baby did not appear dehydrated but as a precaution, the baby was admitted for observation. Nothing abnormal was found, he took his feeds and his stools were normal. His mother took him home 2 days later. When the situation was repeated a few weeks later, this time on a Friday, it seemed a strange coincidence. The doctor sat down with Carl's mother to give her the chance to talk about any problems. She said she was lonely, she had no family nearby and admitted that the baby had not had diarrhoea, but she was desperate to have a break.

Taking the child to the hospital or family doctor may be a cry for help by parents who feel they cannot cope any longer. Hospital is not the best place for the children but with no suitable alternative immediately available, and when parents are at breaking point, the baby is safe and the parents have an opportunity to sort themselves out.

DISADVANTAGED PARENTS

The parents who are least able to cope have limited physical, mental or psychological resources. Their problems may be made worse by unemployment, overcrowding, low income, marital discord, illness of the wife, being a single-parent or having a large family.

Living in poor conditions

The immediate environment in which many disadvantaged families live is often neither pleasant nor safe. Supervision of children playing outside is impossible from the 10th floor flat, so that they either have to play outside unsupervised or be kept indoors where there is inadequate space and limited opportunities for play.

The district may have few facilities such as community centres, sports facilities, parks or playground and school age children wander around, play football in the streets or sniff glue in the cemetery. There may be no child health clinics and sometimes no general practitioner so that a visit to the doctor or clinic may involve a bus ride with a toddler and baby. It is easier and cheaper not to go. The disadvantaged are the least likely to investigate their rights and to seek help.

It is hardly surprising that the children develop more infections, are not immunised and have more accidents. School performance is often poor with little support from parents.

Help for disadvantaged families

During the last decade much has been done to improve the health and standard of living in poor urban areas. The proportion of households without a fixed bath has decreased from 37.6% (1951) to 1.9% (1981). New housing continues to be built and there is a greater awareness of the need for open spaces, playgrounds and facilities for leisure, although not all local councils are willing to spend their limited budgets on these facilities.

Efforts are now being made to concentrate health funds and services on areas of greatest need. General practitioners are encouraged to practise in these areas, child health clinics are set up if none exists and more health visitors may be employed in the area. Informal groups set up in health centres for mothers with young children encourage them to make contact with the health services, as well as providing support, opportunities for meeting others and a break from the home.

Special facilities

In some deprived areas special centres have been set up which the mother and child may attend.

Nursery centres provide day nursery and nursery school facilities, and are open for long hours and all the year round. Parental involvement is encouraged. The child may attend temporarily but most are expected to remain there from the age of joining to school entry.

Some nursery centres include a 'drop-in' centre for parents with young children where, for example, a toy library and facilities for washing clothes may be provided. It provides an opportunity for mothers to meet and have a cup of coffee while the children play, or they can chat while doing their washing. Professional advice is also available.

Family centres aim to help the parents. Both parents and children attend on a daily basis. Programmes are set up to improve, for example, parenting skills and home management and at the same time parents are helped to understand their children's needs better. There may be play sessions where the parents play with their children alongside play therapists.

There are a variety of schemes which arrange for workers to visit the family home where help is needed. The visitor is usually a mature voluntary worker who has had a family and visits as a friend to give support. Having been accepted by the family she gently gives practical tips and makes suggestions on improving the mother's home management and child care. Another type of help involves helping a specific locality rather than individual families by providing extra services and facilities with the necessary staff.

PREPARATION FOR PARENTHOOD

People spend years training to be a plumber, a nurse or a professional singer yet training for parenthood is not considered important or even necessary. Perhaps if it was taken more seriously, there would be fewer parents with unrealistic ideas about their baby's abilities. In the past most girls grew up knowing the capabilities of babies for they had helped to care for the younger children in the family.

There are many sources of information about children and child rearing. Yet very little help is given to a couple to learn about the effects of having a young baby in the house for 24 hours a day. The adaptation of roles, the restrictions on activities, the anxiety and the financial implications all apply to every couple. It would be better if they were aware of these changes in their lifestyle when they were planning to have a baby.

If more organised preparation for parenthood (or childrearing) is advisable, where and when should it begin? At home, school, the youth club, adult evening classes or the ante-natal clinic? At present school lessons are given on child care but other subjects which relate to it, are not integrated with it. Pringle (1980) suggests that an understanding of human psychology and child development must be the foundation for a broadly based programme of preparation for parenthood at school. It should include sex education and personal relationships, family planning, home economics and political education as well as practical experience with young children.

Methods of raising the status of parenthood would benefit children and their parents, as would more facilities for young children whose mothers wish to return to work. Mothers who stay at home to care for their children could be paid an allowance. Parents could be given more support if there were appropiate counselling services. Most of the present services are geared to helping families in a crisis, for example a telephone life-line for a parent who is desperate or a home for battered wives.

REFERENCES AND FURTHER READING

Central Statistical Office 1986 Social trends 16. HMSO, London
Davie R, Butler N, Goldstein H 1972 From birth to seven. A report of the National Child Development Study (1958 cohort) National Children's Bureau. Longman, London
Kempe R S, Kempe C H 1978 Child abuse. Fontana, London
National Children's Bureau Highlight No. 62 1984 Family life—education in secondary schools; review of practice. National Children's Bureau, London
Pringle M K 1980 A fairer future for children. Macmillan, London
Pugh G, De'Ath E 1984 The needs of parents. Macmillan, London

Illness in children today
Measurements of child
  health in the
  community
  Infant mortality rate
Immunisation
Sudden infant death
  syndrome (cot
  deaths)

Accidents
Prevention of accidental
  poisoning
Developing countries
  Reducing the death rate
  and improving child
  health

13

Trends in child health

An emphasis on child health rather than sickness has been encouraged for many years by experts in child care. However, the improvement of social conditions and increase in preventitive medicine do not have the glamorous image and popular appeal of life-saving hospital drama.

More children survive in the UK than formerly and the majority have never been fitter yet the incidence of childhood illness remains high. 50% of all children are admitted to hospital in the first 5 years of life. Diseases which formerly killed or maimed children for life, such as diphtheria and polio, are now prevented by immunisation. Severe infections like tuberculosis are controlled by antibiotics; surgery and other techniques enable many more disorders to be treated, and severe malnutrition is unusual.

ILLNESS IN CHILDREN TODAY

The more common conditions for which children require hospital treatment are:

— congenital defects; serious infections

— injuries resulting from accidents
— conditions related to social problems
— surgery
— intermittent treatment for conditions such as cystic fibrosis
— cancer, for which life expectancy has increased considerably.

Other children who may be well known in the ward and have short spells in hospital, are those with long-term diseases such as asthma, epilepsy, diabetes and physical and mental handicap.

Compared with the comparatively small number of children who require hospital care, the problems in the community are considerably greater. There are increasing numbers of handicapped children requiring care at home with hospital back-up. Psychiatric disorders and behaviour problems are increasing and dental caries is widespread. 27% of children in the UK have already had a general anaesthetic for dental treatment by the age of 8 years. Serious medical problems in older schoolchildren and adolescents are related to alcohol, drugs and glue sniffing. The cycle of deprivation in which disadvantaged families are caught up, is difficult to break out of, and continues from one generation to the next for the majority.

MEASUREMENTS OF CHILD HEALTH IN THE COMMUNITY

How can the standard of child health actually be assessed in a local community or in a country? It is easy to gain an impression of a place in a quick visit, and first impressions may be correct but not always. Generalisations can be misleading and national policies on health and welfare need to be based on facts.

The infant mortality rate has been found to be a sensitive

indicator of a population's health and is used by health workers, politicians and planners in decision making and allocation of funds.

Infant mortality rate (IMR)

The infant mortality rate is the number of deaths under 1 year per 1000 live births. This is an internationally agreed definition so that the rate in different countries or in different regions of the country can be compared. Other measurements which are relevant to child care include the neonatal mortality rate (the number of babies who die within the first 28 days of life per 1000 live births) and the perinatal mortality rate which gives the number of stillbirths and babies who die in the first week of life.

Variations in infant mortality rates

During the 1950s England and Wales had the second lowest IMR in the world but since then it has fallen behind those of other countries (1984 IMR 9.5). The effect of the environment on children's well-being is reflected in the IMR for England and Wales in each social class and also when the figures of different regions of the country are compared.

Classification of social class by occupation

I	Professional
II	Intermediate (most managerial occupations)
III	Non manual and skilled manual
IV	Partly skilled
V	Unskilled

Children in social classes IV and V are more likely to be stillborn or born with a handicap than those in social classes I or II and they are smaller and lighter. These children have more illness, more admissions to hospital and

Table 13.1 Infant mortality rate (England and Wales 1983) by social class

Social class	I	II	III	IV	V
IMR	6.2	7.6	8.6	11.9	12.8

more accidents, but the family receives less medical care and less children are immunised. The children also have lower scores on reading and arithmetic tests at 7 years, and are more likely to be maladjusted. Illegitimate children also have above average rates of morbidity and mortality.

IMMUNISATION

Immunisation is an effective method of reducing illness and death. Many children in the UK are not immunised in spite of advice from doctor and health visitor, posters and advertising campaigns. Yet children die each year from whooping cough and many suffer from the complications of diseases such as measles. 70 900 people, mostly children, developed whooping cough in the epidemic of 1982 and 14 died. After adverse publicity in the 1970s, the immunisation uptake rate for whooping cough fell ·from 80% to 35%. Since then the figure has risen again to about 64%. Immunisation must be seen to be effective and safe and its benefits must out weigh any risk to the individual. The cost to the health service also has to be weighed against the cost of caring for those who would develop the disease.

Whooping cough (pertussis) is an unpleasant disease at any age and the deaths which occur are usually of infants. Infants with whooping cough rarely whoop as older children do, and are more likely to· have apnoeic attacks. They usually require hospital care for constant observation and nursing, and may develop bronchopneumonia. Other complications include convulsions due to asphyxia during spasms of coughing, and intracranial and subconjunctival bleeding.

Vaccination is recommended for all children in the UK taking into account the recommendations of the UK Joint Committee on Vaccination and Immunisation as follows:

Contra-indications to whooping cough vaccine

The vaccine should not be given to children with a history of:

- any severe local or general reaction (including a neurological reaction) to a preceding dose
- cerebral irritation or damage in the neonatal period, fits or convulsions.

Special consideration about the advisability of giving the vaccine is required for those:

- whose parents and siblings have a history of ideopathic epilepsy
- with developmental delay thought to be due to a neurological defect
- with neurological disease.

SUDDEN INFANT DEATH SYNDROME (cot deaths)

Occasionally babies are found dead in their cots. Cot death is the major single cause of death between 1 and 12 months with 1 242 deaths in 1984. The infants are usually under 1 year of age, the majority between 2 and 4 months. The cause is not always known, but in some cases the history reveals symptoms of infection prior to the death which did not appear serious to the parents at the time. The most commonly cited symptoms include undue drowsiness, a cough, 'snuffles', diarrhoea and reluctance to feed. It is thought that one-third of sudden infant deaths could be prevented if symptoms like these were taken more seriously and help sought.

Other causes have been suggested such as overheating, suffocation and allergy. Factors associated with an increased incidence of sudden infant deaths include young mothers, mothers who smoke, illegitimacy, bottle feeding, low birth weight, twin pregnancy and lower social class. When infants assessed as having an increased risk of sudden death have been closely monitored, the incidence of the condition appears to decrease. Monitoring included frequent health checks by health visitors and prompt attention when the babies had minor symptoms or were slightly off colour.

ACCIDENTS

Accidents cause 50% of the deaths of children between 1 and 15 years in the UK. 1 in 5 of all admissions to hospital of this age group is due to trauma. The cost to the child and his parents in suffering and anxiety, and the financial cost to the country, is enormous.

Children who have accidents

It is not unusual for a person to be labelled 'accident-prone' and most people know someone whom the label fits. The accident-prone child may be clumsy, careless, excitable or reckless. Boys have more accidents than girls, and the child's age influences the type of accidents he has.

1- to 4-year-olds are mobile, oblivious of danger and curious. Children have been known to feed their younger sibling in the pram with poisonous berries. Over half the accidents at this age occur in the home.

5- to 9-year-olds are more independent but inexperienced. The child killed in a road traffic accident is most likely to be a pedestrian and most accidents occur outside the home.

Children over 10 years are involved in more road traffic accidents, often bicycling or once they are 16 years old, motor cycling.

Road traffic accidents

These make up one-third of all accidents and half of those who die are child pedestrians. In an environment geared to the motorist, fast moving traffic makes it difficult and dangerous for children to cross roads. Some parents overestimate the ability of their young children, for example in one survey 19% of parents of 2-year-olds thought that their children could safely cross a busy road on their own. The majority of traffic accidents involving children occur in residential areas where a child may run onto the road to retrieve a ball, or run across it without warning.

Urban roads could be made safer by slowing down the traffic but such measures are not popular with the general public, particularly motorists. Children benefit from educational schemes such as the Green Cross Code and cycling proficiency schemes. Parents and the general public could be better educated about the unreliability of children's responses especially when they are engrossed in a game or distracted momentarily.

More public interest has been focused on injuries sustained by car passengers. As a result it is now illegal in the UK to have a child on the knee of the front seat passenger or a child under 12 years sitting in the front seat. Car seats for small children in which the child is restrained are now widely used and attachments are available to hold a carry cot in position. Another group of road users who are at risk of injury are older adolescents on motor cycles. Courses on safety measures and how to ride correctly are organised in most towns.

Burns and scalds

Small children are at greatest risk of being scalded, in fact 75% of scalds occur in children under 5 years. The main causes in order of frequency are liquids in cups or mugs, in teapots, kettles or saucepans.

Often the mug is placed in an apparently safe place such

as on a high table, but the child manages to reach it or to pull the tablecloth underneath it, so that it tips over him. The flexes from electrical equipment such as the kettle or iron are also liable to be within reach of the toddler.

Hot fluids should be out of the toddler's reach and adults should not drink a hot fluid while holding a child. Saucepan handles should be turned towards the back of the stove and a guard fixed round the top of the stove prevents the pans being pulled or knocked over. Fire-proof nightclothes and fires correctly guarded reduce the incidence of burns.

Falls

Children under 5 years suffer a considerable number of head injuries resulting from falls. These are often the result of climbing to explore the environment but also through falling out of windows and off balconies or outside stairways. Some accommodation designed for families appears to have been built without any consideration for children's safety. Windows which swing open can push a child out if he has climbed onto the window sill. Some bannisters are as good as climbing frames and the child may fall onto a concrete stairwell ten floors below. Older children without adequate play or leisure facilities will find entertainment elsewhere, for example playing on derelict property or daring each other to walk along the outer ledge of a railway bridge. Accidents occur in playgrounds where children may misuse equipment or fall onto a hard surface. Falls in the home may be due to poor upkeep of the building so that a window with a broken catch can be opened by small children. The baby may fall when he is left lying unattended on his parents' bed while his mother answers the doorbell.

Poisoning

Although death from poisoning is rare in childhood, the incidence of ingestion of poison is extremely high. About

Table 13.2 Commonest substances ingested by children (survey 1981, Nottingham)

Substance	% of children
Medicines	33.3
Turpentine	21.3
White spirit	
Household cleaners	21.3
Plants	13.3
Cosmetics	6.6
Alcohol	4.0

16 000 children are admitted to hospital each year with suspected poisoning and many more are seen in casualty departments and at doctors' surgeries. Toddlers choose strange substances to eat in the home and they are most likely to do this at a time of family stress. Examples of substances ingested are bleach, rat poison, lipstick, paint remover and contraceptive pills.

Treatment

The child requires urgent attention. The priorities are to find out what has been taken, to induce vomiting (in most cases) and to observe the child for the effects of the poison. The parent is asked to take the container and the remains of any substance suspected of being swallowed to the hospital with the child, so that it can be identified. Vomiting is induced unless the poison is corrosive or volatile or the child is unconscious. A corrosive substance will continue to burn any tissue which it touches, and volatile substances (petrol, paraffin, turpentine and turpentine substitute) give off fumes which may be inhaled and cause further lung damage. The child who has taken a corrosive substance is given plenty of water to drink. For all other poisons vomiting in induced by giving a dose of syrup of ipecacuanha. If this is not effective a gastric washout is performed. Depending on the effect of the drug and the amount taken, the child is admitted to hospital for observation.

Drugs which are found in many homes and are particularly dangerous for children are aspirin, iron and antidepressants.

Aspirin (salicylates)

This group includes aspirin tablets and Oil of Wintergreen. One teaspoonful of this oil can be fatal.

Clinical signs of salicylate poisoning are nausea, vomiting, tinnitus, fever and dehydration, hyperventilation and hypoglycaemia or hyperglycaemia.

Iron

A small child may be fatally poisoned by as little as 2 g of iron. The early signs of poisoning are gastrointestinal symptoms and gastrointestinal bleeding. During the period 8–16 hours after ingestion, the child seems better. He may then collapse, become comatose and have fits.

Antidepressant drugs

Amitriptyline and imipramine are some of the most dangerous drugs consumed by children.

Clinical signs: respiratory and cardiovascular depression, fits, dilated pupils, loss of consciousness, atropine-like effects, cardiac arrhythmias.

PREVENTION OF ACCIDENTAL POISONING

As most cases of accidental poisoning occur in the home and involve drugs, steps have been taken to reduce the number of these accidents. Child-resistant containers have been introduced and some tablets are now packed in 'blister packs'. Eating tablets packed in this way takes time and effort, and the child is more likely to be found before he has eaten too many. Poison informations centres have been set up so that medical staff can obtain information at any time about an unusual substance which has been ingested.

Safety measures in the home

- Keep all medicines in a locked cupboard with internal and external medicines separated.
- Do not leave tablets or containers around the house.
- Do not transfer tablets from one container to another.
- Dispose of unused drugs by returning them to the chemist or flushing them down the lavatory.
- Teach children not to take tablets or medicine unless given to them by parents.
- Keep bleaches, cleaning agents and soap powders in a locked cupboard in the kitchen.
- Keep all poisonous substances in the garage or garden in a locked area or on a high shelf, out of children's reach.
- Always keep poisonous substances in a clearly-labelled securely fastened container.
- Teach children about poisons in the home and about poisonous plants and berries.

Another suggestion is that doctors should prescribe drugs in smaller amounts so that there are less drugs in the house.

Educating the public

Although the rate of poisoning has been reduced by measures already taken, the number of children poisoned and of accidents generally could be reduced dramatically if the public were more aware of the risks and how to reduce them.

Individuals can be given information when they come in contact with medical or nursing staff, for example the family doctor, the health visitor, the antenatal clinic or the child welfare clinic. The health visitor may visit the child's home after he has been treated in hospital for poisoning. Many parents are more interested in accident prevention at this time, and accept advice readily. Written information or a printed leaflet given to a mother helps to reinforce verbal advice and may be useful at a later date.

Television advertisements and series on accident prevention for adults and children are valuable teaching aids. Mothers (and fathers) also learn from magazine articles. Some shops who sell children's clothes include information about safety in their catalogues. Information about accident prevention may be given to groups of people in discussion, talks, videos or films. Participants might be playgroup leaders, a school class, nurses, policemen or mothers' groups. However information is useless unless people can be persuaded to listen and act on it, and if this could be achieved, the incidence of child poisoning in the UK would drop dramatically.

DEVELOPING COUNTRIES

Although the UK infant mortality rate could and should be improved there is no comparison between it and the rates in developing countries. Of the 10.3 million infant deaths world-wide, 0.3 million occur in the developed world and 10 million in the developing world.

Table 13.3 Examples of varying infant mortality rates (1982)

Rate	Country	IMR
Over 100	Sierra Leone	200
43 countries	Malawi	170
	India	120
26–100	Morocco	100
33 countries	Iraq	70
	Yugoslavia	30
25 or less	Italy	13
30 countries	UK	11
	Sweden	7

Politics, social change and culture

The influence of these factors on children's health are as relevant in the developing world as they are in the UK. Aid for a needy country may be withheld by other countries because of political differences and within a country, one tribe or group of people may be victimised by their own government.

Population growth, natural disasters which may be partly man-made, wars and movement of large numbers of refugees from one area to another, all contribute to poor conditions and shortages already existing. It is estimated that almost 1000 million people are trapped in the circle of poverty, malnutrition, disease and despair. This saps people's energy, reduces work capacity and limits their ability to plan.

Cultural and tribal customs may be beneficial, for example prolonged breast feeding of the infant. However, it is not easy to persuade people to change customs which are not beneficial, such as applying cow dung to the newborn baby's umbilical cord.

Childhood illness in developing countries

Many infant deaths occur at birth or in the first week of life, and these are due to mothers being malnourished, numerous pregnancies with short intervals in between, and inadequate antenatal and obstetric care.

After this period, the child's ill health and risk of dying are closely related to the environment. In poor communities infection is rife as a result of unclean drinking water, un-hygienic sanitation, overcrowding, ignorance about hygiene, and lack of facilities. The child's resistance to infection is reduced by factors such as malnourishment and intestinal parasites. Episodes of infection, occurring every few weeks, sap the child's energy and reduce his reserves, making him more susceptible to the next infection. As a result, growth and development are retarded and those who survive may be left with a mental or physical handicap.

Reducing the death rate and improving child health

A scheme involving four low-cost and simple methods of saving children's lives is being promoted by the United Nations Children's Fund (UNICEF), which could halve the children's death rate in the world. Its effects are already beginning to be apparent in some areas. The four methods are:

— oral rehydration therapy administered by the mother
— monthly weighing of all children and the use of a simple child growth chart
— the promotion of breast feeding
— immunisation.

Oral rehydration therapy

Diarrhoeal dehydration is the biggest single killer of children in the world. It is estimated that around 4 million die each year from this condition. Oral rehydration therapy is being used in several countries and has proved to be an effective method of reducing the serious effects of diarrhoeal illness.

The treatment

A glucose-salt mix is given orally by the mother to her child at home. The solution is made up by mixing a powder, supplied in individual packs, with a litre of drinking water. It contains potassium and bicarbonate as well as glucose and salt, and is recommended by UNICEF and WHO. Small quantities are given every few minutes and the amount required to correct the dehydration (measured by the glassful) in a given time is explained on a simple chart.

As a home remedy to prevent dehydration or where packages of powders are not available to treat it, parents are taught to make their own solution. A small two-ended plastic measure is used to teach the correct quantities, approximately a teaspoonful (5 ml) of sugar and the tip of the spoon of salt, which are added to a glass of water. The solution must always be tasted before it is given and should not be more salty than tears.

In 1984 it is estimated that half a million children were saved by this therapy, at a time when less the 15% of the world's families were using the technique. The number of children requiring hospital care and intravenous therapy was reduced dramatically. The long-term prevention of diarrhoea depends on education, improved water supplies, sanitation and hygiene, but in the meantime oral rehydration is a valuable method of preventing deaths due to diarrhoea.

Monthly weighing

The value of monitoring the child's weight on a centile chart is that the growth curve identifies problems early. A gradual deterioration in weight gain due to malnutrition may start to develop a year or more before clinical signs appear, so that early treatment can be given in the home.

Promotion of breast feeding

Breast feeding protects the baby from the worst effects of poverty — malnutrition (generally) and gastroenteritis. It is recommended until the child is 2 years old: an additional advantage of prolonged breast feeding is that it is a useful method of birth control. The baby's diet should be supplemented by food from 4–6 months of age.

Immunisation

5 million children in the developing world die each year due to six infectious diseases which could be prevented by immunisation. The diseases are measles, diphtheria, pertussis, polio, tuberculosis and tetanus. Most nations of the

world, WHO and UNICEF are all working to make immunisation against these diseases available to all children by 1990.

It is apparent from what has already been said, that the main causes of death in childhood in the developing world are very different from those in developed countries. Conditions such as marasmus (calorie starvation) and kwashiorkor (protein deficiency) are major causes of children's deaths but in many more instances malnutrition is a contributory factor. The deaths of 2 million children who die annually as a result of measles are rarely caused solely by the disease. Rather, it is the final blow to a malnourished child who is weakened by frequent infections of various types, from which he does not fully recover before he develops another. The combination of malnutrition and childhood infections such as whooping cough or measles can be deadly. If the scheme promoted by UNICEF is successful world-wide, this combination will cease to be a problem.

REFERENCES AND FURTHER READING

Bewley B 1986 The epidemiology of adolescent behaviour problems. British Medical Bulletin 1986 42(2): 200–203

Central Statistical Office 1986 Social trends 16. HMSO, London

Davie R, Butler N, Goldstein H 1972 From birth to seven. A report of the National Child Development Study (1958 cohort) National Children's Bureau, London

Grant J P G 1984 The state of the world's children 1985. Oxford University Press for UNICEF, Oxford

Jackson R H 1977 Children, the environment and accidents. Pitman, Tunbridge Wells

Morley D 1973 Paediatric priorities in the developing world. Butterworths, London

Office of Population Censuses and Surveys (OPCS) Mortality statistics DH3 85/3

Sadler J 1972 Children and road safety, a survey among mothers. OPCS Social Survey. HMSO, London

Survey of children's dental health (United Kingdom 1983) 1985 HMSO, London

Appendix

Calculating dosages

CALCULATING THE VOLUME OF A STOCK SOLUTION REQUIRED FOR A CHILD'S DOSE USING THE FORMULA

This section gives a more detailed explanation of the calculations in Chapter 7 as well as some examples to test yourself. Common errors with fractions and decimals are included for those who need revision.

If you had difficulty with the calculation in the text, work through this section as it is written. From the beginning, use the formula and write down your calculation each time, even though the arithmetic is very easy. This will enable you to work out the more difficult ones later which cannot be calculated in your head.

The formula

$$\frac{\text{strength required}}{\text{strength available}} \times \text{volume of stock dose} = \frac{\text{volume}}{\text{required}}$$

Example: ampoule of pethidine 50 mg in 1 ml
dose prescribed   20 mg

Using the formula, this becomes

$$\frac{20 \text{ (strength required)}}{50 \text{ (strength available)}} \times 1 \text{ ml} = \text{volume required (ml)}$$

$$= \frac{20}{50} \text{ which cancels down to } \frac{2}{5} \text{ or } 0.4 \text{ ml}$$

Now check your answer mentally. Does it seem reasonable considering the strength of the stock solution? ½ ml would contain 25 mg. 0.4 ml is just under half, so it is what we would expect.

Remember! The volume of the stock dose must always be included.

Test 1 (Answers on p. 314)

1.1 Oral Vallergan elixir 42 mg is ordered as a premedication. The bottle contains 6 mg in 1 ml. How much would you give?

1.2 A dose of 24 mg is required from a stock solution containing 40 mg in 2 ml. How much is required?

1.3 Atropine 150 micrograms is ordered for a baby's premedication. The ampoule contains 600 micrograms in 1 ml. How much is given?

If any of your answers were incorrect, re-read the initial example and try again. Check that:
— the formula was correct
— the figures were correctly placed in the formula
— your arithmetic was correct.

Common errors in the arithmetic

Multiplying a fraction

When multiplying a fraction by a whole number only the

figure above the line is multiplied, and not the figure under the line.

Cancelling down a fraction

When cancelling down (reducing the fraction to the lowest denominator) both the figure above the line and the figure below the line must be divided by the same number.

Question 1.1: cancel down by 6

$$\frac{42}{6} = \frac{7}{1} = 7$$

Question 1.3: $\dfrac{150}{600} = \dfrac{15}{60} = \dfrac{3}{12} = \dfrac{1}{4}$

Converting a fraction into a decimal

Divide the figure above the line by the figure below the line

Example: $\dfrac{3}{5} = 5\overline{\smash)3.0} = 0.6$

If any answer remains incorrect after checking the formula and your arithmetic, consult your tutor.

Test 2 (Answers on p. 314)

Now that you have grasped the formula, work through these calculations. Notice that as they become more difficult, it is impossible to calculate them in your head.

2.1 Strength of stock solution: 5 mg in 1 ml.
     Dose required: 2 mg.

2.2 A pethidine ampoule contains 50 mg in 1 ml.
     Dose required: 40 mg.

2.3 Strength of stock solution: 0.5 mg in 1 ml.
Dose required: 0.4 mg

2.4 From stock of digoxin elixir 0.05 mg in 1 ml.
Dose required: 0.01 mg.

2.5 An antibiotic is made up with 250 mg in 2 ml.
The baby requires 62.5 mg.

Check your answers and go carefully through the formula steps or arithmetic workings if any are incorrect.

Possible difficulties

Decimal point

Make the calculation easier by getting rid of the decimal point whenever possible. You can do this by multiplying both the figure above the line and the figure below the line by the same number.

Example: (Question 2.3): multiplying both figures by 10

$$\frac{0.4}{0.5} \times 1 = \frac{4}{5} \times 1 = \frac{4}{5} = 0.8 \text{ ml}$$

Here, by multiplying the figures above and below the line by 10 (moving the decimal point 1 column to the right), the decimal point is removed. Sometimes multiplying by 100 (moving the decimal point 2 columns to the right) is necessary.

Example (Question 2.4): multiplying both figures by 100

$$\frac{0.01}{0.05} \times 1 = \frac{1}{5} = \frac{1}{5} \text{ ml} = 0.2 \text{ ml}$$

Remember! When doing a written calculation, always place the figures under each other in their correct columns (100s, 10s, 1/10ths). The position of the decimal point is then clear and you are much less likely to make a mistake when moving the decimal point, which could be a fatal error.

Example (Question 2.5):

$$\frac{62.5}{250} \times 2 = \frac{125}{250} = \frac{25}{50} = \frac{1}{2} = 0.5 \text{ ml}$$

In this instance the easiest method for most people is to remove the decimal point by multiplying the figures above the line first. There is often more than one method of calculating the answer — use the easiest one for you.

Test 3 (Answers on p. 314)

3.1 Omnopon 8 mg is required from an ampoule containing 20 mg in 1 ml. How much would you give?

3.2 Pethidine ampoules contain 100 mg in 2 ml. How much is required for an adolescent who is prescribed 60 mg?

3.3 Strength of stock solution 0.6 mg in 1 ml.
Dose required for an infant is 0.15 mg. How much is given?

3.4 Digoxin elixir contains 0.05 mg in 1 ml. How much is required to give 100 micrograms?

Possible errors

Question 3.2

You may have forgotten to include the volume of the stock dose.

Question 3.3

When multiplying both figures by 100 (to dispose of the decimal point) you may have omitted a '0' below the line thereby making 0.6 into 6 instead of 60.

Difficulties with different units of weight

The prescription and the stock solution should always be in the same unit of weight (gram, milligram or microgram). Occasionally they are not, as in Question 3.4. All students should be familiar with the metric system and SI units. The important units in this context are:

1 gram (g) = 1000 milligrams (mg)
1 milligram = 1000 micrograms

Question 3.4

A dose of 100 micrograms is required from a stock solution containing 0.05 mg in 1 ml.
The calculation must be worked out in the same unit, so the first step is to convert both figures to the same unit. It is usually calculated in the smaller of the units to avoid fractions.

Calculation
0.05 mg = 0.05 × 1000 micrograms
        = 50 micrograms

The calculation now becomes $\frac{100}{50} \times 1 = 2$ ml

The major safeguards against giving an incorrect dose are:

- two people always check and give the drug
- each one calculates the amount and then they compare notes
- difficult calculations are worked out on paper
- always check mentally that the amount seems reasonable.

ANSWERS

1.1 7 ml
1.2 1.2 ml
1.3 0.25 ml
2.1 0.4 ml
2.2 0.8 ml
2.3 0.8 ml
2.4 0.2 ml
2.5 0.5 ml
3.1 0.4 ml
3.2 1.2 ml
3.3 0.25 ml
3.4 2 ml

Glossary

Anaemia
thalassaemia, spherocytosis and sickle cell anaemia are all inherited haemolytic anaemias.

Biliary atresia
congenital absence of bile ducts, causes obstructive jaundice from early infancy.

Bronchiectasis
chronic condition of the lungs in which bronchi and bronchioles are dilated, usually caused by repeated chest infections. Rare nowadays.

Cervical adenitis
inflammation of the lymph glands in the neck.

Circumcision
excision of the foreskin (prepuce) of the penis, performed for religious or medical reasons. Bleeding is a complication of surgery.

Cleft lip and palate
abnormality develops in early fetal life. 25% of children have cleft lip, 25% have cleft palate, 50% have

both. Surgery for lip at 3 months and for palate around 1½ years.

Coeliac disease a disorder of malabsorption caused by intolerance to gluten, the protein in wheat and rye. Diagnosed in young children from time of weaning. Cured by gluten-free diet for life.

Coarctation of aorta a narrowing of the aorta which in severe cases causes heart failure in infancy. Blood pressure is higher in arms than in legs. Treated successfully by surgery.

Cystic fibrosis recessively inherited disease in which secretions of exocrine glands are abnormally viscid. It causes meconium ileus, malabsorption and repeated chest infections. Daily treatment required for life, most die in late teens or early adult life.

Fallot's tetralogy a congenital abnormality of the heart with pulmonary stenosis and the root of the aorta displaced over a hole in the intraventricular septum, resulting in an enlarged right ventricle. The child is cyanosed. Can be corrected surgically.

Haemophilia a sex-linked recessively inherited bleeding disorder, due to deficiency of Factor VIII in the blood. Bleeding may be spontaneous or due to injury, treated by IV injection of cryoprecipitate (Factor VIII). Home treatment has revolutionised children's lives.

Henoch Schönlein purpura a generalised disorder causing purpuric rash, pain and swelling of joints, abdominal pain, malaena and haematuria. Steroids may be given. Occasionally causes permanent renal damage.

Hiatus hernia a congenital laxity of the oesophageal hiatus which causes vomiting in infancy. Treated by nursing the infant in the sitting position, thickening the feeds and possibly giving antacids before feeds.

Hirschsprung's disease caused by absence of parasympathetic ganglia in distal part of large bowel, causing intestinal obstruction in neonate or chronic constipation in the child. Treatment is surgical.

Hydrocephalus an increased amount of cerebrospinal fluid (CSF) in the brain, due to defect in outflow of CSF. In infancy, the head enlarges and the fontanelle bulges. Treated by insertion of 1-way valve to drain excess fluid away.

Imperforate anus low type of ano-rectal agenesis. The anus of the newborn baby is not patent. Corrected by minor surgery.

Inguinal hernia during its descent into the scrotum the testis is accompanied by a pouch of peritoneum, the processus vaginalis, which normally closes during infancy. Both inguinal hernia and hydrocele are caused by patent processus vaginalis which is ligated if it persists.

Intussusception an invagination of bowel into an adjacent distal segment causing small bowel obstruction in children under 2 years. Sudden attacks of screaming, caused by abdominal pain, occur in a previously healthy baby. Urgent treatment is required to avoid necrosis of the bowel as a result of obstruction.

Meckel's diverticulum a remnant of a duct which arises from the ileum in fetal life and may persist as a diverticulum. It may become inflamed, or the adjacent bowel may bleed or perforate.

Meconium ileus intestinal obstruction in the neonate which occurs in 10% of children with cystic fibrosis. Small bowel obstruction is caused by thick viscid meconium. Treatment is usually surgical.

Microcephaly a head which is below the normal range in size. Usually associated with mental handicap.

Muscular dystrophy Duchenne's muscular dystrophy, a sex-linked recessive disorder, is the commonest type. Symptoms occur by the age of 5 years, and boys are confined to wheelchairs by their teens.

Nephritic syndrome acute nephritic syndrome previously called acute nephritis, often precipitated by streptococcal throat infection. There is a sudden onset of haematuria, oliguria, proteinuria, oedema and hypertension.

Nephroblastoma   a malignant tumour arising from primitive kidney cells which occurs in young children. Treated with cytoxic drugs, surgery and radiotherapy. Prognosis is good for many children.

Neuroblastoma   a malignant tumour arising from sympathetic nervous tissue. It is usually highly malignant.

Oesophageal atresia   an interruption in the lumen of the oesophagus often associated with a tracheo-oesophageal fistula. Surgery is performed in first week of life.

Orchidopexy   the operation of bringing undescended testes into the scrotum.

Osteomyelitis   infection of the bone which usually affects long bones. Treated with high doses of intravenous antibiotics and sometimes surgery. There are serious complications if it is neglected.

Patent ductus arteriosus   a congenital abnormality. The fetal blood vessel (from pulmonary artery to aorta) which by-passes the lungs remains patent after birth. Corrected surgically.

Patent processus vaginalis   see inguinal hernia.

Perthes' disease   necrosis of the head of the femur which occurs mostly in boys between 4 and 8 years. Treated by resting the joint (no weight bearing) for a prolonged period or by surgery.

Phenylketonuria   a recessively inherited disease caused by the inability to metabolise phenylalanine. Treated by a strict diet. The untreated child becomes severely mentally handicapped and all babies (UK) are screened for the condition at birth.

Pyloric stenosis   hypertrophy of the pyloric muscle, commonest in male babies between 3 and 6 weeks. It causes projectile vomiting after feeds and the baby is hungry. Loss of weight and dehydration occur if treatment is delayed.

Rheumatoid arthritis   sometimes called Still's disease. These are several types of juvenile chronic arthritis, from single painful joints to a generalised disorder. Steroids are used with caution because of their side effects.

Scabies   a contagious disease causing a very itchy rash. Mites' burrows in the skin appear as irregular grey lines with a black dot at the end. A papular rash and scratch marks may be present. Treated by application of lotion to whole body.

Talipes   A congenital abnormality of the foot. There are several types, one being club foot. Treated by manipulation, splinting and sometimes surgery.

Transposition of the great vessels   A congenital heart defect in which the aorta and pulmonary artery are transposed so that the aorta arises

from the right ventricle. Cyanosis and
heart failure develop in infancy. Can
be corrected surgically.

Undescended testes in fetal life the testes descend from
high in the abdominal cavity to the
scrotum. Orchidopexy is performed
by 3 years if the testes have not
descended.

Index

Note: Page numbers in italics denote Glossary entries.

Abused child *see* Child abuse
Accidents, 147, 295, **297–303**
  burns and scalds, 298–299
  falls, 299
  in hospital, 147, 149
  prevention, 298–299, 301–303
  road traffic, 298
  see also Poisoning; Safety
Administration, 8, 18, 20, 71, 73, 77,
      289
  central government, 8, 18, 20
  local government, 71, 73, 77, 289
Admission to hospital, **17–18, 57–62,**
      183–186, 262–264
  assessment and history taking,
      57–62
  emergency, 18, 59
  hearing-impaired child, 183–185
  planned, 17, 263
  pre-operative, 263–264
  preparation of child for, 262–263
  visually handicapped child,
      185–186
Adolescent, 34–40, 79, 115–118,
      131–139, 197, 251–253, 293
  development, 115–118
  handicapped, 34, 131–139,
      251–253
  in hospital, 34–40
  long-term illness, effects of, 34,
      36–40
AIDS, 88

Alcohol, 79, 88, *293*
  adolescent and, 79, 88, 293
  fetal development, effect on, 88
Anaemia, *315*
Analgesics *see* Pain, child in
Anatomy and physiology, 3, 167, 221
  body fluid, % of weight, 221
  immune system, 3, 167
  kidney, infant's, 221
  respiratory tract, 3, 167
Antenatal care, 88, 119, 122
Anxieties, parents', 17–18, 21, 35, 48,
      51, 137, 164, 166, 261–262,
      274–277
Apnoeic attacks, 168–169
Assessment of child, 57–62, 121–122
  developmental, 121–122
  nursing process, 57–62
  under 5 years, 121–122
Asthma, 56, 170–172, 293
  see also Long-term illness
Auto-immune deficiency syndrome
      see AIDS

Baby *see* Infant
Barrier nursing *see* Infection
Bathing child and infant *see*
      Cleansing, personal
Battered child *see* Child abuse
Bed wetting *see* Enuresis
Biliary atresia, *315*

Blind child see Visually handicapped child
Blood pressure, 232–233, 236
Body water, percentage of weight, 221
Bonding, 21, 23, 94–96
Bowels, 104–105, **228–230,** 260
  see also Diarrhoea
Breathing, 166–179
  administration of drug by nebuliser, 172
  assessment and problems of, 167–171
  infant, 167–170, 175–178
  oxygen therapy, 173–175
  rates, respiratory, 167–168
  see also Cardiac arrest; Croup
Bronchiectasis, 315
Bronchiolitis, care of baby with, 175–178

Calculation of drug dosages, 149, **152,** 308–314
Cardiac arrest, 155–158
Case conference see Child abuse
Catheterisation, urinary, 234
Centile chart see Growth
Cerebral palsy, 133–137, 251–253
Cervical adenitis, 315
Child abuse, 94, 124–125, 130, 219–221, **281–286**
  at risk register, 130, 286
  background, 94, 125, 282–283
  case conference, 286
  hospital care of abused child, 219–221, 284–286
  nurses' feelings, 285
  parents, 220–221, 283, 285
  types of, 281–282
Child development see Development, child
Child health, 292–307
  developing countries, 303–307
  mortality rates, 293–295, 303–304
  see also Community, child health in
Child in hospital, 4, 6–45
  adolescent, 34–40
  behaviour, 23–24, 26, 28–30, 35, 40–43

individualised care see Patient assignment
  infant, 23–28
  observation of, 15–16
  pre-school child, 24–28
  schoolchild, 28–34
  separation from mother, 4, 22–28
  see also Admission to hospital; Nursing sick children; Parents
Childminder, 71–72
Chronic illness see Long-term illness
Circumcision, 315
Cleft lip and palate, 315
Cleansing, personal, and dressing, 238–251
  bathing, child, 245–246
  dress in hospital, 239, 246
  infant care, 239–241, 243–245
  see also Mouth care; Skin; Teeth
Coarctation of aorta, 316
Coeliac disease, 316
Combined home and hospital care, 50–51, **261–262**
Comforter (cuddly), 61, 103
Communicating, 74–75, 180–190
Community, child health in, 18, 54–55, **119–139,** 286, 289, 292–303
  clinics, child health, 119, 289
  health visitor, 18, 54–55, 119–126, 297
  mental handicap nurse, 137–139
  midwife, 119, 122
  primary health care team, 119
  school health service, 126–133, 286
  see also Handicapped child; Environment
Congenital abnormalities, 81, **87–88,** 320
Consent for operation, 143, 264
Constipation, **229–230,** 260
Convulsions (fits), 16, 164–166
  febrile convulsions, 164–166
  infant, 16
Cot death, 296–297
Court Report, 8, 77
Croup (laryngotracheobronchitis), 170, 178–179
Cuddly see Comforter

Culture, influence on child, 74–76, 304
  diet, 76
Cystic fibrosis, 287, 293, *316*
  see also Long-term illness

Day care, hospital *see* Nursing sick children
Deafness *see* Hearing-impaired child
Death, 44–45, 272–278
  care of dying child, 44–45, 275–277
  child's ideas on, 272–273, 276
  explanations, 273–274, 275–276
  helping the family, 45, 274–277
  nurses' feelings, 44–45, 276
  siblings, 276–278
  see also Mortality rates
Defects, congenital *see* Congenital abnormalities
Dehydration, 223, 226–228, 305
Dental care *see* Teeth
Deprivation, **74,** 219–221, 293, 304
  see also Child abuse
Developing countries, 303–307
  environment, 304
  mortality rates, 303
  improving health, 305–307
Development, child, 4–5, 26, 28, 30–31, 35, 61, **89–118,** 180–181, 220, 304
  birth–1 year, 92–101
  1–2 years, 101–106
  2–4 years, 106–108
  4–7 years, 109–112
  7–12 years, 112–115
  adolescence, 115–118
  delay in, 4, 90, 220
  milestones, 89, 97, 99, 102
  language, 97, 99–100, 103, 180–181
  regression in, 5, 26, 28, 30–31, 35, 61
Diarrhoea, care of child with, 223, **226–228,** 305–306
Diet *see* Eating
Disadvantaged families, 74, 78, **288–290,** 293–295
  see also Deprivation
Discharge from hospital, 28, 271

Discipline, 40–43, 78
  in ward, 40–43
  in society, 78
Dislocation of hip, congenital, 4, 62–64, **261**
District nursing sister, 119
Divorce, effect on child, 69, 79
Doctor, 12, 119, 125–133, 276–277
  hospital, 125, 128, 276–277
  in community, 119, 125
  school, 126–133
Dressing (clothing) *see* Cleansing, personal and dressing
Drinking, 62–63, **221–228,** 270–271, 305–306
  assessment and problems, 62–63, 221–223
  oral rehydration therapy, 305–306
  reluctance to drink, 62–63, 222–223, 270–271
Drugs, 15, 79, 88, **149–154,** 293, 299–303, 308–314
  administration of, 15, 149–154
    infants and toddlers, to, 151
  calculations of drug dosages, 149, 152, 308–314
  injections, 153–154
  poisoning by *see* individual item
  society, problem in, 79, 88, 293
Dummies *see* Mouth care
Dying child *see* Death

Eating, 205–221
  assessment and problems, 213–216
  see also Infant feeding
Eczema, 247–251
  care of child with, 248–251
Educational psychologist, 127
Eliminating, 104–105, **228–237,** 260
  assessment and problems, 229–232
  bowels, 228–230, 260
  toilet training, 104–105, 228–229
  urine, 228–234, 236–237
Enteritis *see* Diarrhoea
Environment, 67–71, 77, 90, 123–124, 286–290, 298, 304
  community, 77, 288–290, 298
  developing countries, 304

Environment (*contd*)
home, 67–71, 90, 123–124,
286–287
see also Nursing sick children;
Safety

Emotional needs, 4, 6, **22–26**, 61, 282,
285–287
see also Deprivation; Development
Enuresis (bed wetting), 26, 123–124,
133
Erikson, E, **96**, 105
Explanations to child concerning
hospital, 38–39, 42–43, 262–263
surgery, 33, 39, 263–265
treatment, 31–33, 38–39, 150, 153,
199–201
visiting, 21–22, 27–28

Failure to thrive, 219–221
Fallot's tetralogy, *316*
Family, 18, 21, 27, 29, 31, 59, 61,
67–88, 92, 282–288, 294–295
influence on child, 59, 61, 74–80,
92, 282–288, 294–295
one parent family, 18, 69, 287–288
parents' role in, 67–71
role in care of sick child *see* Parents,
role in ward
Fears and fantasies, child's, 17, 24–26,
28–33, **108**, 200–201
in hospital, 17, 24–26, 28–33,
200–201
young child, 108
Febrile convulsions *see* Convulsions
Feeding, infant *see* Infant feeding
Fetal development, factors affecting,
87–88
Fits *see* Convulsions
Fluids *see* Drinking
Fontanelles, anterior and posterior, **93,**
223, 270
Freud, S, 98, **105**

Gastroenteritis *see* Diarrhoea
Genetics, 80–87
chromosomes, 82

counselling, genetic, 84–85
genes, 83
patterns of inheritance, 84
Growth, 36, 39, **89–96**, 129–130,
216–217, 304
centile charts, 129–130, 216, 306
height and length measuring,
216–217
see also Failure to thrive; Weight

Haemophilia, *316*
Handicapped child, 113, 125–126,
131–139, 251–253, 293
assessment, 131, 133–135, 138–139
district handicap team, 134
health visitor, role in care, 56–57,
125–126
home care, 133–139, 215–216
infant, 133
key worker, 135
mentally, 134, 137–139, 161
community mental handicap
nurse, 137–139
training programmes, 134, 138
paediatric assessment unit, 134
parents of, 136–137
physically, 55, 113, 134, 198–199,
215–216, 252–253
feeding, 215–216
play, 55, 113, 134, 198–199
positioning, 198, 252–253
schooling, 131–132, 135–136
see also Long-term illness
Head lice *see* Infested head
Health education, 120–124, 129–130,
132–133, 246, 290, 296, 298,
302–304, 306
and health visitor, 120–124, 302
in schools, 129–130, 132–133
in society, 290, 296, 298, 302–304,
306
see also Safety
Health visitor, 18, 54–55, **119–126**, 302
Hearing impaired child, 61, 181–185
deafness, degrees, 181–182
in hospital, 181–185
Height and length *see* Growth
Henoch-Schönlein purpura, *317*
Hiatus hernia, *317*

Hip, congenital dislocation *see*
    Dislocation of hip, congenital
Hirschsprung's disease, 230, *317*
Hydrocephalus, 262, *317*
Hypothermia *see* Temperature, body

Immobilised child, 253–256,
    260–262
  bed, in, 253, 260–261
  combined home and hospital care,
    261–262
  restraint, methods of, 256–259
  traction, in, 253–256, 260–261
Immunisation (vaccination), 61,
    119–120, 123, 126–127,
    295–296, 306–307
  programme (UK), 120, 127
Imperforate anus, *317*
Infant (baby), 51, 156–162, 167–169,
    177, 216, 243–245, 247,
    256–259
  bathing and hygiene, 243–245
  feeding *see* Infant feeding
  holding during investigations, 51,
    256–259
  length, measuring, 216
  mouth care, 177, 247
  resuscitation, 156–157
  respirations, 167–169
  temperature, 158–162
    recording, 161–162
  weight, measuring, 216
  see also Child in Hospital;
    Development; Drugs,
    administration of; Infection,
    cubicle nursing; Mortality rates
Infant feeding, 98, **205–211,** 213–214,
    304, 306–307
  artificial (bottle), 205–209
    feeds, preparation of, 208
  breastfeeding, 205–207, 306
  problems related, 213–214
  weaning, 98, 209–211
Infection, ward, 15, 147–149,
    227–228
  barrier nursing, 148–149, 227–228
  cubicle nursing (reverse barrier),
    147–148

Infested head, 129–130, 132, 241–242
  treatment of, 242
Inguinal hernia, *317*
Inherited disorders *see* Genetics
Intravenous infusion, 224–226
  differences from adults, 224
  observation of child, 226
Intussusception, *318*
Investigations, 170–172, 233–234,
    256–259
  ear examination, 171
  holding child for, 256–259
  nasal swab, 172
  sputum specimen, 170
  throat swab, 171–172
  urine specimen, 233–234
  venepuncture, 27, 256–257

Language, development of, 97,
    99–100, 103, **180–181**
  see also Speech
Laryngotracheobronchitis *see* Croup
Liaison health visitor, 54–55
Long-term illness, 30, 34, 36–40,
    136–137, 261–262, 287, 293

Malabsorption, 219, 229
Measles, 120, 306–307
Meckel's diverticulum, *318*
Meconium, 92, 229
  ileus, *318*
Meningocele *see* Spina bifida
Microcephaly, *318*
Midwife, 119, 122
Milk, constituents of, 207
Mobilising, 251–262
  assessment and problems, 252–256
  see also Immobilised child
Module, paediatric, 5, 10
Moro response, 94–95
Mortality rate, infant, 88, **293–295,**
    303–304
  neonatal and perinatal rates, 88,
    294
  perinatal mortality rate, 294
Mouth care, 239, 246–247
  daily teeth cleaning, 239, 246

Mouth care (contd)
  dummies, 239, 246
  of sick child, 246–247
  mouth toilet, 247
Muscular dystrophy, 318
Myelomeningocele see Spina bifida

NAI see Child abuse
Napkin rash, 240–241
Nasogastric tube, 214–215, 218–219
  feeding, 214–215, 218–219
    procedure, 218–219
  passing, 218
National Association for the Welfare
  of Children in Hospital
  (NAWCH), 8
National Society for the Prevention of
  Cruelty to Children see NSPCC
Nebuliser, use of, 172
Neglect see Deprivation
  see also Child abuse
Neonate (newborn), 158, 160, 167,
  221, 294, 304
  immunity, 167
  kidney function of, 221
  mortality rate, 294, 304
  temperature control in, 158, 160
Nephritic syndrome, 318
Nephroblastoma, 318
Nephrotic syndrome, 234–237
  care of child with, 235–237
Neuroblastoma, 319
Nightmares, 26, 28, 43–44
Non-accidental injuries see Child
  abuse
NSPCC, 73, 284, 286
Nurse, student, 5, 13–16, 38
Nursery, day, **72**, 289–290
Nursery nurse, 52–53
Nursing process, 57–63
Nursing sick children, 3–16, **22–45,**
  47–56, 62
  history of, 6–10
  home care, 8, 56, 261–262, 287
  in hospital, 3–16, 22–45, 47–56
    day care, 56
    difficult situations, 40–45
    patient assignment see individual
     item

  ward environment, 6–15, 31
  ward team, 47–55
  planning care, 56, 62

Obesity, 128
Oedema, 232
  see also Nephrotic syndrome
Oesophageal atresia, 319
Ointment, application of, 247
One-parent family, 18, **69,** 79,
  287–288, 295, 297
Oral rehydration therapy see Drinking
Orchidopexy, 319
Osteomyelitis, 319
Oxygen therapy, 173–175

Paediatric assessment unit see
  Handicapped child
Pain, 27, 33, 51, 153, 188–190
  assessing, 188–189
  painful procedures, 27, 33, 51, 153,
    189–190
  relieving, 189–190
  see also Death
Parents
  in ward,
    advice re visiting, 8, 18–19,
     20–22, 27–28, 35
    anxieties of, 17–18, 21, 35, 51
    facilities for residents, 19–20
    help required, 20, 23–24, 48–49,
     220–221
    role, 12–13, 17–18, **48–52,** 178,
     261–262, 274–277
  role in family, 67–71
Parenthood, preparation for, 290–291
Patent ductus arteriosus, 319
Patent processus vaginalis see Inguinal
  hernia
Patient assignment (patient
  allocation), 24, 27, 31, 59, 227
Pediculosis capitis see Infested head
Perinatal mortality rate see Mortality
  rates
Perthes' disease, 319
Pertussis see Whooping cough
Phenylketonuria, 320
Piaget, J, **105,** 108, 111, 115

Place of Safety Order, 284
Planning care *see* Nursing sick
  children
Platt Report, 8
Playgroup, 73
Playing, 13, 33–34, **191–202**
  birth–1 year, 192, 196
  1–3 years, 192–193, 196
  3–5 years, 193–196
  5–12 years, 196–197
  explaining treatment through,
    199–200
  hospitals (doctors and nurses),
    200–201
  in hospital, 13, 197–202
  see also Development; Toys
Playleader, 55
Poisoning, 218, **300–303**
  by antidepressants, aspirin and iron,
    301
  emergency treatment, 218, 300
  prevention, 301–303
Postoperative care, 267–271
  airway, maintaining, 267, 269
  observations, 267, 269–270
  wound care, 267
Pre-operative care, 33, 39, 143, 200,
    262–266, 268–269
  consent for anaesthetic and surgery,
    143, 264
  explanations, 33, 39, 199–200,
    263–265
  preparation for admission, 262–263
Pre-school child, 71–74, 106–111,
    193–196
  see also Child in hospital; Day care
Pressure sores, 254–255, **260,** 262
  preventive measures, 254, 260
Primary health care team, 119
Primitive reflexes, 93–94
Psychiatric disorders, 293
Puberty, 115
Pulse, 168, 270
  rates by age, 270
  recording, 168, 270
Pyloric stenosis, *320*
Pyrexia, 162–166
  care of child with, 162–164
  febrile convulsions, 164–166

Registered Sick Children's Nurse
    (RSCN), 10, 47–48
Respiratory arrest *see* Resuscitation
Respiratory rates, by age, 168
Restraining the child, 256–259
  types of restrainer, 258
Resuscitation, 155–158
Rheumatoid arthritis, *320*
Rickets, 75
Robertson, J, 24
Roden, J, 33
Rubella (German measles), **87–88,**
    127

Safety
  at home, 122, 288, 298–299,
    301–303
  in children's ward, 143–158
    procedure after accident, 147
Scabies, 239, 320
School, 53–54, 72, 126–133,
    135–136, 202–203
  hospital, 53–54, **203**
  normal, 126–133, 135–136, **202**
  nursery, 72
School health service, 126–133
  dentist, 126, 130–131
  doctor, 126–127, 130–131, 133
  nurse, 126–133
Schoolteacher, 53–54, 109, 113,
    130–131, 133–134, 203
  home tutor, 134
  hospital, **53–54,** 203
  normal school, 109, 113, 130–131,
    133
Scoliosis, 128–129
Screening tests, 127–129
  hearing, 127
  phenylketonuria, *320*
  scoliosis, 128–129
  vision, 127–128
Siblings, 21, 29, 31, 276–278
Single-parent family *see* One-parent
    family
Skin, 239–251
  assessment and problems, 239–242
  irritable, 247–250
  lesions, types of, 239–240
  napkin rash, 240–241

Smoking, 88, 297
Social class, **294–295,** 297
Social problems, 18, 61, 74, 123–125, **281–291**
  related to hospital admission, 18, 74, 286–287
  see also Disadvantaged families
Social worker, 61, 119, 125, 127, 137, 264
Society, 77–80, 302
  changes in, 77–80
Speech, 131, 180–184
  communicating with deaf child, 181–184
  therapist, 131
  see also Development, language
Spina bifida, 262
Stools, 92, **229–230**
Stridor, 170
Sudden infant death *see* Cot death
Surgery *see* Pre- and postoperative care

Talipes, *320*
Teaching parents, 23, 48, **50–51,** 166, 289, 305
Teeth, 130–131, 239, 246, 293
  cleaning, 239, 246
  dental caries, incidence, 293
  dental inspections, school, 130–131
  eruption of first teeth, 239
  see also Mouth care
Television, 79–80
Temperature, body, 158–166
  hypothermia, 158, 160
  infant, 158–162
  recording, 160–162
Temper tantrums, 43, 106–107

Toddler, 71–74, **101–108,** 121–122, 192–193
  see also Child in hospital
Toilet training, 104–105, 228–229
  see also Enuresis
Tonsillectomy, 268–271
Toys, 11, 31, 119
  library, 119
  see also Development; Playing
Traction, 4, 62–64, 254–256
  care of child on, 260–261
  observations of, 254
  Gallow's, 255–256
Transposition of great vessels, *320*

Undescended testes, *321*
Urine, 228–234
  micturition, young child, 231
  normal volumes, 231
  specimens, obtaining, 233–234
  see also Toilet training

Vaccination *see* Immunisation
Visually handicapped child, 185–186
  blindness, degrees of, 185
  in hospital, 185–186
Vitamins, 75, 211

Warnock Report, 135
Weaning *see* Feeding
Weight, 96, 216, 232
  centile charts *see* Growth
  measuring child's, 216, 232
  measuring infant's, 216
Whooping cough (pertussis), 120, 123, 169, **295–296,** 306
Wound, care of, 267–268